Small Animal Dermatology

The What's Your Diagnosis? Series

What's Your Diagnosis? is an exciting new series of short books that combine problem-based learning, case studies, and questions and answers.

The books are entirely case based, with theory, background and analysis interwoven into each case. Questions are used to test the reader's knowledge in identifying signs, underlying differential diagnoses, diagnostic plans and treatment options. Answers are then provided to guide the reader through the rationale for the choices made.

Other What's Your Diagnosis? Series Titles

Small Animal Ophthalmology: What's Your Diagnosis?

By Heidi Featherstone and Elaine Holt

978-1-405-1-5161-0

Canine Internal Medicine: What's Your Diagnosis?

By Jon Wray

978-1-118-9-1816-6

Small Animal Dermatology

What's Your Diagnosis?

Jane Coatesworth, M.A., Vet.M.B., Cert.V.D., MRCVS
Animal Health Trust, Lanwades Park, Kentford, Newmarket, Suffolk, UK

WILEY Blackwell

Registered Office
John Wiley & Sons, Inc., 111 River Street, Hoboken, NJ 07030, USA

Editorial Office
111 River Street, Hoboken, NJ 07030, USA

For details of our global editorial offices, customer services, and more information about Wiley products visit us at www.wiley.com.

Wiley also publishes its books in a variety of electronic formats and by print-on-demand. Some content that appears in standard print versions of this book may not be available in other formats.

Library of Congress Cataloging-in-Publication Data

Names: Coatesworth, Jane, 1964- author.
Title: Small animal dermatology : what's your diagnosis? / Jane
    Coatesworth.
Description: Hoboken, NJ : John Wiley & Sons, Inc., 2019. | Series: What's
    your diagnosis? | Includes bibliographical references and index. |
    Identifiers: LCCN 2018051416 (print) | LCCN 2018053074 (ebook) | ISBN
    9781119311140 (Adobe PDF) | ISBN 9781119311126 (ePub) | ISBN 9781119311119
    (paperback)
Subjects: | MESH: Skin Diseases–veterinary | Animals, Domestic | Skin
    Diseases–therapy | Differential Diagnosis | Case Reports
Classification: LCC SF992.S55 (ebook) | LCC SF992.S55 (print) | NLM SF 901 |
    DDC 636.08965–dc23
LC record available at https://lccn.loc.gov/2018051416

Cover Design: Wiley
Cover Images: Courtesy of Jane Coatesworth

Set in 10/12.5pt MinionPro by SPi Global, Chennai, India
Printed and bound in Singapore by Markono Print Media Pte Ltd

10 9 8 7 6 5 4 3 2 1

Contents

Acknowledgements

My grateful thanks and heartfelt appreciation for the love and counsel of my family and friends, and for the kindness and support of many past and current colleagues at the Animal Health Trust.

Abbreviations

ACTH	adrenocorticotropic hormone
ALP	alkaline phosphatase
ALT	alanine aminotransferase
AN	acanthosis nigricans
APTT	activated partial thromboplastin time
ASIT	allergen specific immunotherapy
BAER	brain auditory evoked response
CAFR	cutaneous adverse food reaction
CDA	colour dilution alopecia
CLE	cutaneous lupus erythematosus
DLE	discoid lupus erythematosus
DMSO	dimethyl sulfoxide
EL	epitheliotropic lymphoma
ELISA	enzyme-linked immunosorbent assay
GABA	gamma-aminobutyric acid
GGT	gamma-glutamyltransferase
H&E	haematoxylin and eosin
HAC	hyperadrenocorticism
HCS	hepatocutaneous syndrome
IBD	inflammatory bowel disease
IgE	immunoglobulin E
IgG	immunoglobulin G
MCP	mucocutaneous pyoderma
PARR	PCR for antigen receptor rearrangements
PAS	periodic acid Schiff
PCR	polymerase chain reaction
PF	pemphigus foliaceus
PT	prothrombin time
SA	sebaceous adenitis
SAM-e	S-adenosyl-L-methionine
SCT	Sertoli cell tumour
SLE	systemic lupus erythematosus
SLIT	sublingual immunotherapy
TCT	thrombin clot time
TSH	thyroid stimulating hormone
UCCR	urine cortisol: creatinine ratio
UDS	uveodermatologic syndrome
VCLE	vesicular cutaneous lupus erythematosus

Introduction

Dermatology is an interesting area of clinical practice. The skin is the largest organ of the body and is continually renewing itself. The skin is influenced by diet, hormones and systemic disease and colonised by bacteria, yeasts and parasites. Despite this variety of interactions, the skin has limited responses to insult and so many skin diseases present with a similar appearance.

Dermatology cases account for around 30% of the case load of small animal first opinion practice. It is important to aim for a definitive diagnosis at an early stage, otherwise cases can be given a series of reactive symptomatic treatments and remain a source of frustration for both vets and owners. Many cases, such as those with allergic skin disease, are controllable but cannot be cured. A realistic prognosis, owner education, financial estimates, owner motivation and an appropriate treatment plan all follow from a definitive diagnosis.

It is very helpful to maintain the discipline of a systematic approach. A well-rehearsed systematic approach to history taking and physical examination will ensure that important information is not missed when we are tired, busy or distracted. This is followed by noting down a list of the problems. A problem list is not included in the cases in this book as the section heading gives the main presenting problem such as pruritus, alopecia and so on. The History sections are edited to contain only the pertinent points, in contrast to the usual 20 pages of history that may accompany a skin case. Following the problem list, it is very important to develop a list of differential diagnoses. This is a list of possible diseases that fit the history and clinical signs and the list forms the basis on which diagnostic tests are selected. It is helpful to list the differentials in order of likelihood, as this can save time and money when performing diagnostic tests. A disease that is not on the differential list may not be looked for, so time spent creating a good differential list is very helpful and gives structure and direction to the case work-up. Readers in different geographical areas will have different differential lists, or the same list in a different order, to reflect local prevalence of disease.

Itch scores are referred to in some of the cases in this book. A score of 1/10 is a normal dog with an occasional scratch or lick at the skin and 10/10 is an animal showing almost continuous pruritic behaviour. Asking owners to allocate an itch score to their pet can be helpful in gauging relative pruritus levels. The score is very subjective, but the same owner scoring over time can add useful information to the overall picture. Inviting owners to point to a visual analogue scale has been shown to be more representative than conjuring a number from their thoughts.

Clinicians are problem-solving detectives with good abilities to analyse and filter large amounts of information. This book is designed to enhance clinical problem-solving skills and can be approached as a series of mini challenges. The text details the process of clinical decision making using real cases from first and second opinion practice. The book contains a variety of case material from the UK, from the common to the rare. It is not intended to be a comprehensive textbook, but covers the broad range of dermatology discussed in the 34 cases that have been included.

Further reading

Hill, P.B., Lau, P., and Rybnicek, J. (2007). Development of an owner-assessed scale to measure the severity of pruritus in dogs. *Veterinary Dermatology* 18: 301–308.

Alopecia

Alopecia is an obvious clinical sign and is frequently of concern to owners. The hair coat can play an important part in the relationship between owner and pet by affecting the way the animal looks and feels. The presence of hair protects the underlying skin from physical, chemical and ultraviolet damage and plays a role in thermoregulation. There is often a wide range of possible causes of alopecia and identifying the specific cause can be challenging. Alopecia can be the result of congenital or hereditary abnormalities in hair growth, endocrine disease, allergic skin disease, hair follicle death, parasites and fungal or bacterial infections.

The term alopecia refers to an abnormal absence of hair, which can be partial or complete. The term hypotrichosis is used for an abnormal diffuse thinning of the hair coat. A sparse hair coat is a normal feature of some locations, such as between the ear and eye of a cat. Glabrous skin is innately very sparsely haired or devoid of hairs. The extent of glabrous skin is breed dependent but typically occurs at the axillae, ventral abdomen and concave aspects of the pinnae. Certain breeds have extensive genetically determined areas of alopecia that are considered to be normal, examples include the Mexican Hairless dog (Xoloitzcuintli), the Chinese Crested dog and the Sphynx cat.

Alopecic cases can be usefully divided into those with inflammatory skin lesions and pruritus, and those with non-inflammatory skin lesions and no pruritus. The history and clinical examination can help to place a case in one of these two groups. Examples of inflammatory and pruritic skin conditions include allergic skin disease, ectoparasitic disease with a hypersensitivity component, and surface or superficial bacterial or yeast infections. Conditions with non-inflammatory primary skin lesions include the endocrine diseases and follicular dysplasias. Clinicians need to be alert for secondary bacterial or yeast infections, which may complicate many of the non-inflammatory conditions and result in focal inflammation and pruritus.

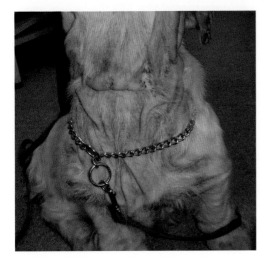

Figure A.1 Shows the ventral neck of a young Clumber Spaniel. There is marked erythema, and extensive self-inflicted alopecia from persistent rubbing and scratching. The dog has atopic dermatitis and a secondary *Malassezia* dermatitis.

Small Animal Dermatology: What's Your Diagnosis? First Edition. Jane Coatesworth.
© 2019 John Wiley & Sons, Inc. Published 2019 by John Wiley & Sons, Inc.

Non-inflammatory alopecia is often associated with abnormalities in the hair growth cycle. Thyroid hormone is important in triggering the active growth phase (anagen), consequently dogs with untreated hypothyroidism have an increasing number of hair follicles arrested in telogen. High levels of glucocorticoids or oestrogens can also cause telogen arrest by delaying the onset of anagen. Telogen hairs are eventually shed from the follicles and there is no new hair growth to replace them.

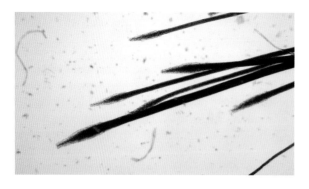

Figure A.2 Shows a group of plucked hairs from a dog with hypothyroidism. The hair bulbs are all in telogen, the resting phase of the hair growth cycle. Telogen hairs have a characteristic narrow and pointed 'spear shaped' root end.

Pattern alopecia is a non-inflammatory and non-pruritic condition that has a symmetrical pattern and is seen in certain breeds, most notably the Dachshund. The caudal thighs, convex aspects of the pinnae, ventral abdomen, thorax and chest are the commonly affected areas. The hairs and hair follicles become progressively miniaturised and then stop growing, leaving areas of permanent alopecia. Pattern alopecia is first seen in young adult dogs and has a slowly progressive course. It is a cosmetic condition with no associated pruritus or systemic signs.

Post clipping alopecia is an abnormal delay in hair regrowth after clipping. This can occur in any breed, but is more common in plush coated dogs. Plush coated dogs, such as the Nordic breeds, make a significant investment of resources into growing their dense coat. The hairs grow to a fixed length and are then retained in the resting phase (telogen) over a long period of time before being replaced. Clipping a plush coated dog during the long resting phase can lead to a prolonged period of alopecia before new hair regrows. The reason for the delayed anagen is not understood, but it may take up to 2 years for the alopecia to be replaced with a new hair coat.

The hair follicle has a very high level of metabolic activity at the time of new hair production, and is nourished by a plentiful blood supply. Interruptions to the blood supply can result in local ischaemia and the death of hair follicles. The resulting well-defined areas of scarring alopecia are usually permanent. Ischaemic dermatopathies, with clinical signs of scarring alopecia, include dermatomyositis and local reactions to rabies vaccination. Dermatomyositis is most often seen in the Shetland Sheepdog and Collie breeds, and is a heritable condition.

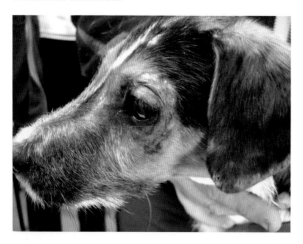

Figure A.3 Shows the left face of a young adult Jack Russell Terrier. There is a well demarcated alopecic ring surrounding the left eye. The dog is not pruritic and the lesions do not appear to be inflamed. There are similar lesions around the right eye, on the margins of the ear pinnae and at the tip of the tail. Skin biopsies demonstrate a vasculitis/vasculopathy but the inciting cause is unclear. No further lesions occur, but there is persistent alopecia over a 9-year period of follow up.

Alopecia can occur after inflammation and damage to the hair follicle; for example, in dermatophytosis, demodicosis or bacterial folliculitis. The damage can also be immune mediated; for example, the attack of hair follicles mediated by cytotoxic lymphocytes in alopecia areata. Hair follicles can be damaged by extremes of temperature; for example, the scarring alopecia associated with thermal burns and hot or freeze branding.

Alopecia in cats is often self-induced. The abrasive tongue, combined with persistent over-grooming behaviour, can produce extensive hair loss in a relatively short period of time. It can be more challenging in cats to decide if the alopecia is self-inflicted, as owners typically spend less time observing a cat in comparison to a dog. Examination of plucked hairs is often helpful to show whether hair shafts have been fractured by self-trauma.

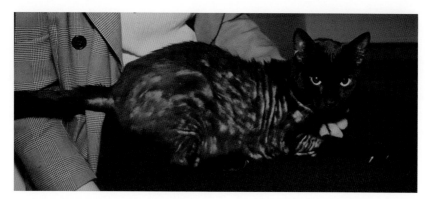

Figure A.4 Shows the right side of a black cat. There is extensive hypotrichosis over the trunk, the proximal tail and proximal hind limbs. The head, distal limbs and distal tail have a normal dense hair coat. This cat has a bilaterally symmetrical self-induced hypotrichosis, resulting from the over grooming associated with a flea bite hypersensitivity.

Skin biopsy can be a helpful diagnostic tool for cases presenting with alopecia. Biopsies should be taken from the centre of an alopecic area so that the histopathologist can identify and assess well established changes. The presence of bacterial and *Malassezia* infections can mask the primary pathology, so it is helpful to control these secondary changes before taking biopsies.

History

A 6 year-old male neutered Airedale Terrier is presented with an 8-month history of hair loss.

The dog is from a rehoming charity and has lived with the owners for the past 3 years. Hair loss was first noticed 8 months ago, starting over the tail head and extending cranially to the lateral body walls, progressing down the hind limbs and most recently involving the neck. He eats, drinks and urinates a normal amount, but is less keen to exercise than usual. The owners have noticed that other male dogs are attracted to their dog in the park. They try to mount him, or to lick his penis. He tolerates this for a short while and then growls and rebuffs them.

Questions

1. Describe the abnormalities and pertinent normal features in Figures 1.1 and 1.2.
2. What differential diagnoses should be considered for this presentation?
3. What tests could you perform to make the diagnosis?

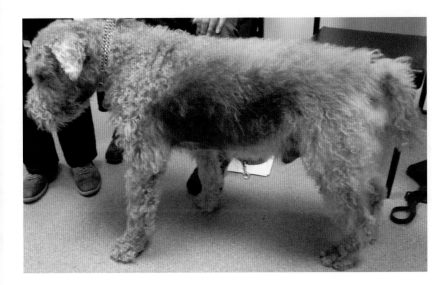

Figure 1.1

Small Animal Dermatology: What's Your Diagnosis? First Edition. Jane Coatesworth.
© 2019 John Wiley & Sons, Inc. Published 2019 by John Wiley & Sons, Inc.

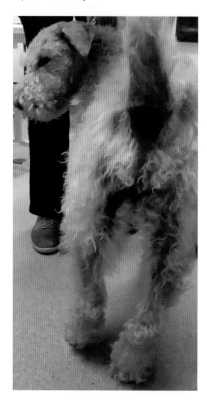

Figure 1.2

Answers

1. What the figures show

Figure 1.1 shows the left side of the dog. There is an extensive area of alopecia on the left body wall with intense hyperpigmentation of the skin. This pattern is repeated on the right side of the dog. The remaining hair coat has an abnormally soft, sparse, pale coloured and woolly appearance, except for the paws and head, which retain a more normal type of coat. The prepuce is drooped.

Figure 1.2 shows the dog from behind. There is alopecia and marked hyperpigmentation of the caudal and medial aspects of the proximal hind limbs, ventral tail and perineum. The remaining hair coat, above the hocks, is sparse and soft.

2. Differential diagnoses

Given the appearance of the skin lesions the following conditions should be considered:

Causes of non-pruritic, bilaterally symmetrical alopecia

- Hypothyroidism
- Hyperadrenocorticism (HAC)
- Cyclic flank alopecia (Airedale Terrier is a predisposed breed)
- Sex hormone alopecia
- Demodicosis
- Dermatophytosis

Causes of the hair coat alterations

- Hypothyroidism
- HAC
- Sex hormone alopecia

3. Appropriate diagnostic tests

Physical examination reveals a grade 3–4 systolic cardiac murmur. There is moderate enlargement of the mammary glands.

Hair plucks show no *Demodex* mites.

Haematology shows a low red blood cell count of 5.22×10^{12} l^{-1} (5.55–8.5×10^{12} l^{-1}) with a normal mean corpuscular volume (normocytic) and a normal mean corpuscular haemoglobin content (normochromic). This mild non-regenerative anaemia could be associated with chronic neoplasia and/or inflammation, or with early bone marrow dysfunction. Hyperoestrogenism, associated with some testicular tumours, can cause initial stimulation of the bone marrow. There is an elevated white blood cell count 21.2×10^9 l^{-1} (6–18×10^9 l^{-1}), elevated bands 1.7×10^9 l^{-1} (0–0.5×10^9 l^{-1}) and an elevated segmented neutrophil count 13.99×10^9 l^{-1} (4–12×10^9 l^{-1}). The leukocytosis, neutrophilia and a regenerative left shift are indicative of persistent function of the myeloid lineage in the bone marrow and are commonly associated with acute infection, tissue damage or inflammation. Chronic exposure to elevated oestrogen levels can result in significant bone marrow damage and manifest as anaemia, neutropenia and/or thrombocytopenia.

Serum biochemistry shows hypercholesterolaemia 11.2 mmol l^{-1} (3.6–7 mmol l^{-1}). Total T4 and thyroid stimulating hormone (TSH) assays are not tested at this time as, despite the dog being middle aged, lethargic and hypercholesterolaemic, there is a higher index of suspicion of a sex hormone imbalance. Moreover, this dog has chronic disease, which can lead to thyroid panel results being outside of the normal range despite the thyroid gland having a normal capacity.

Urine cortisol: creatinine ratio (UCCR). This test has a high sensitivity and a low specificity for HAC. It is ideal for ruling out HAC when, as in this case, there is a low index of suspicion for the disease. A UCCR within the normal range confidently rules out HAC (here 17.5×10^6, a normal ratio is below 30×10^6). An elevated ratio would need to be further investigated with a low dose dexamethasone suppression test, or an adrenocorticotropic hormone (ACTH) stimulation test, as it may indicate HAC or other non-adrenal related illness.

Abdominal ultrasonography, performed conscious, shows a greater than 10 cm diameter complex mass in the mid-abdomen. The mass is well vascularised and contains multiple cystic structures. The medial iliac lymph nodes are enlarged, slightly heterogeneous and measure around 1 cm in diameter. This may represent local metastasis or reactive local lymphadenopathy. No abnormalities are seen in the liver or spleen. The prostate is mildly enlarged but retains a normal bi-lobed shape. The mass is presumed to be a retained testicle, but a second testicle could not be identified during the ultrasound examination. Atrophy of the contralateral normal testicle is a common occurrence.

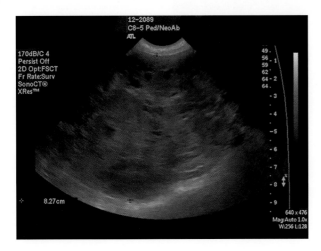

Figure 1.3 Shows an ultrasound image of the abdomen. There is a complex mass, of more than 10 cm diameter, in the mid-abdomen. The mass contains multiple anechoic areas.

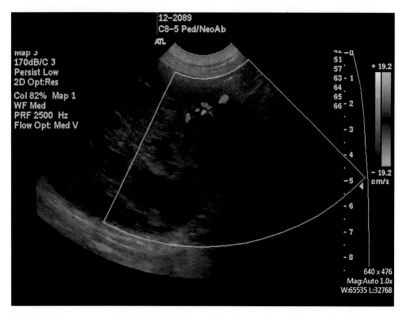

Figure 1.4 Shows a colour Doppler image of the same mass. The colour flow signal indicates that the mass has a well-developed vascular system.

Diagnosis

Probable hyperoestrogenism, associated with a retained testicle that has undergone neoplastic transformation.

Treatment and outcome

Exploratory laparotomy reveals a large and highly vascular mass. The mass is presumed to be a retained testicle and is removed from the mid-abdomen with careful ligation of the substantial blood supply. The second testicle is not found. One local lymph node is excised.

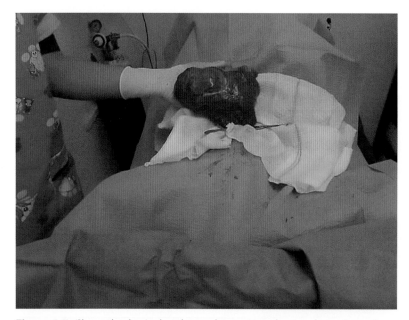

Figure 1.5 Shows the dog in dorsal recumbency, at exploratory laparotomy. A large soft tissue mass, found in the mid-abdomen, is exteriorised but is still attached. The mass is multi-lobulated, and highly vascular.

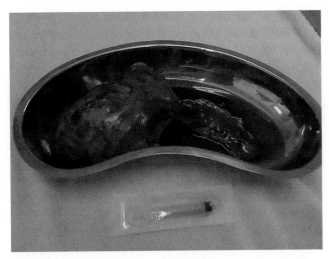

Figure 1.6 Shows the excised mass, with a section of attached vasculature on the right. The 20 ml syringe in the foreground gives an impression of scale.

Histopathological examination of the excised mass shows it to be a retained testicle, containing both a mixed Sertoli cell tumour (SCT) and a seminoma. More than one type of primary tumour in a single testicle is not uncommon. The local lymph node shows reactive change, with no evidence of tumour metastasis. Metastasis is uncommon in SCTs and rare in seminomas and interstitial cell tumours.

The dog recovers well after surgery, and gradually becomes more active and playful. There is progressive hair regrowth at the previously alopecic areas. The new hair is dense, lustrous, darker in colour and has a more robust texture than the previous hair coat.

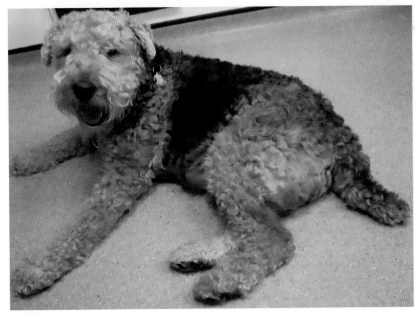

Figure 1.7 Shows the dog 5 months after initial presentation. He has a brighter demeanour and extensive hair regrowth of a normal Airedale-type hair coat. There are marked changes in the colour, density and texture of the hair coat.

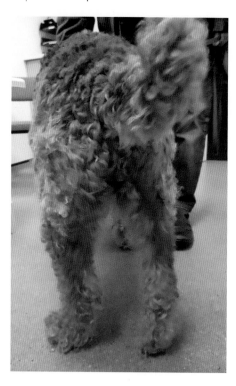

Figure 1.8 Shows the dog from behind, 5 months after initial presentation. There is complete hair regrowth at the previously alopecic areas.

Prognosis

The prognosis is good if the primary tumour is completely excised and no tumour metastasis has occurred. The dog had no apparent oestrogen-induced myelotoxicity.

There is a risk that the other testicle will undergo neoplastic transformation. Up to 50% of dogs have bilateral tumours. The other testicle is presumably also retained, but could not be located for removal during the exploratory laparotomy.

Discussion

This dog has a feminisation syndrome caused by hyperoestrogenism. A male dog may overproduce oestrogen from a neoplastic testicle, or from excessive adrenal gland activity. A female dog may show hyperoestrogenism associated with cystic ovaries, or by over medication with oestrogen. Oestrogen supplementation is most commonly dispensed for urinary incontinence.

General clinical signs associated with hyperoestrogenism are gynaecomastia, a pendulous prepuce, prostatic enlargement, being attractive to male dogs and vulval swelling. Bone marrow suppression is potentially life threatening.

Dermatological signs associated with hyperoestrogenism include bilaterally symmetrical alopecia. This classically starts caudally, especially involving the perineum, and progresses cranially and ventrally. The alopecic areas, as in this case, are hyperpigmented and there is no primary pruritus. A pathognomic dermatological sign, present in this case but not photographed, is a line of erythema and hyperpigmentation between the prepuce and the perineum. So-called linear preputial erythema is uniquely associated with the presence of a testicular tumour and is a useful dermatological marker of internal disease.

Testicles initially develop near the kidney. They usually move through the inguinal ring and are often palpable in the normal scrotal position by 3 months of age. Testicles can be retained at any stage of this journey. The tendency to be cryptorchid is inherited as an autosomal recessive trait, although the Airedale Terrier is not recognised as a breed predisposed to this condition.

Three main types of tumour can develop within testicles – SCTs, seminomas and interstitial (Leydig) cell tumours. The three types occur with approximately equal frequency, usually in the older dog. There is a higher incidence of SCTs and seminomas in retained testicles, but not of interstitial cell tumours. It is likely, in this case, that oestrogen was being produced by the SCT rather than by the seminoma. About one-third of SCTs produce sex hormones, while only a small percentage of seminomas and interstitial cell tumours are functional. Functional SCTs and seminomas tend to produce oestrogens, while functional interstitial cell tumours produce androgens.

Tumour development is likely to be appreciated more quickly in an external testicle than in a retained testicle. The size and shape of the affected testicle is often distorted. Palpation ± ultrasound examination, with comparison to the contralateral testicle, is usually helpful in a descended pair. This dog was adopted from a rehoming charity at 3 years of age as an apparently neutered male. It seems that the history of his undescended testicles was lost at some stage.

Anti-Müllerian hormone (AMH) may be a useful biomarker for cryptorchidism. AMH is produced by the ovaries and by Sertoli cells in the testicles. Correctly neutered animals would be expected to have no measurable hormone. This ELISA test was not employed in this case as there were highly suggestive clinical signs and the abdominal mass was easily found on ultrasound examination.

Further reading

Hayes, H.M. and Pendergrass, T.W. (1996). Canine testicular tumours: epidemiological features of 410 dogs. *International Journal of Cancer* 18: 482–487.

Holst, B.S. and Dreimanis, U. (2015). Anti-Müllerian hormone: a potentially useful biomarker for the diagnosis of canine Sertoli cell tumours. *BMC Veterinary Research* 11: 166.

Lawrence, J.A. and Saba, C.F. (2013). Chapter 28: Tumors of the male reproductive system. In: *Withrow and MacEwen's Small Animal Clinical Oncology*, 5e (ed. S.J. Withrow, D.M. Vail and R.L. Page), 557–561. Maryland Heights, MO: Elsevier Saunders.

Weaver, A.D. (1983). Survey with follow up of 67 dogs with testicular Sertoli cell tumours. *Veterinary Record* 113: 105–107.

History

A 3 year-old male neutered Italian Spinone is presented with an 8-month history of hair loss. Hair loss was first noticed over the dorsal muzzle, the hair subsequently regrew in this area. Hair loss over the dorsum has been slowly progressive with time. The proximal tail is the most recent area to be affected. The dog has an itch score of 4/10, characterised by rubbing against the furniture, rolling on the dorsum and dragging the ventrum along the ground. The degree of pruritus waxes and wanes, and is associated with the presence of visible skin lesions, described by the owner as 'crusty circles'. The owner feels that they refill the water bowl more frequently than normal, but it is unclear which of the three dogs in the house may have an increased water consumption.

Routine vaccinations have not been given since primary inoculations as a puppy. The second dog in the household, a Bassett Hound, is also pruritic. The third dog in the household, another Spinone, does not have any skin issues. All of the dogs have regular anthelmintics and flea control during the summer months.

Questions

1. Describe the abnormalities and pertinent normal features in Figures 2.1–2.4.
2. What differential diagnoses should be considered for this presentation?
3. What tests could you perform to make the diagnosis?

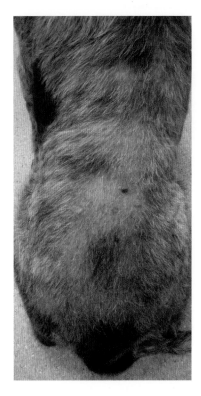

Figure 2.1

Small Animal Dermatology: What's Your Diagnosis? First Edition. Jane Coatesworth.
© 2019 John Wiley & Sons, Inc. Published 2019 by John Wiley & Sons, Inc.

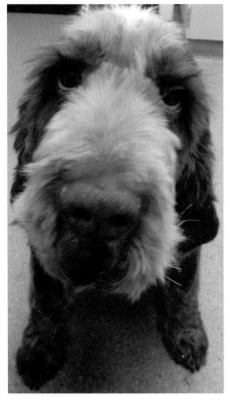

Figure 2.2

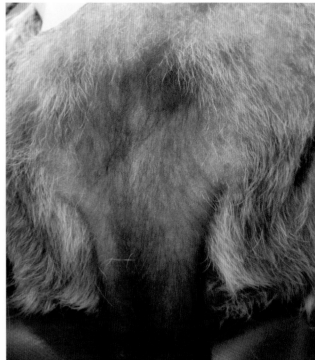

Figure 2.3

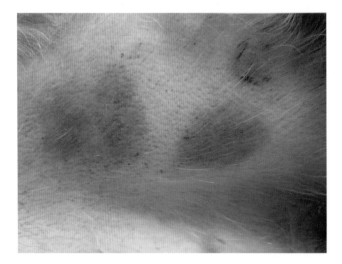

Figure 2.4

Answers

1. What the figures show

Figure 2.1 shows the caudal dorsum from above. There is extensive hypotrichosis over the dorsum and rump. Both grey and brown hairs are affected. The distal tail, at the bottom right of the picture, maintains a normal appearance.

Figure 2.2 shows the dog's face, with a placid and sleepy expression.

Figure 2.3 shows the caudal dorsum and proximal tail. There is extensive hypotrichosis. The exposed skin has a darker skin tone than normal, probably associated with exposure to ultraviolet light. There are no signs of inflammation or excoriation.

Figure 2.4 shows an area of thinly haired skin on the ventral abdomen. There are three hyper-pigmented macules. The two on the right are sharply demarcated. The older macule, on the left, is fading and has a less distinct margin. Note the relatively pale skin tone of the surrounding skin, in comparison to the dorsum in Figure 2.3. The macules are post-inflammatory changes, at the site of previous epithelial collarettes. There is an epithelial collarette, with central erythema and a peeling edge, at the top right of the photograph.

2. **Differential diagnoses**

Given the appearance of the skin lesions the following conditions should be considered:

Causes of alopecia due to pruritus and self-excoriation

- Flea bite hypersensitivity. The dorsum, particularly the caudal dorsum, is a commonly affected area for dogs and cats with this condition. The dog is part of a multi-pet household and flea control is only given in the summer.
- Food intolerance.
- Atopic dermatitis. This dog has onset of clinical signs at less than 3 years of age, lives mostly indoors and has recurrent bacterial skin infections. However, the distribution of affected areas – dorsal muzzle and dorsum – is not typical for atopic dermatitis. The owner was unsure what level of pruritus was present when no 'crusty circles' were seen. This piece of information is very helpful for deciding whether the condition underlying the recurrent pyoderma is pruritic, for example atopic dermatitis, or non-pruritic, for example hypothyroidism.
- Bacterial superficial pyoderma.
- *Malassezia* dermatitis.

Causes of alopecia that are non-pruritic, when uncomplicated by secondary infection

- Hypothyroidism
- Hyperadrenocorticism
- Dermatophytosis
- Demodicosis

3. **Appropriate diagnostic tests**

Cytology. Direct impression smears, from beneath the peeling edge of epithelial collarettes, show neutrophils with intracytoplasmic cocci and are diagnostic of a superficial bacterial pyoderma. Other findings consistent with superficial bacterial pyoderma are: the owner description of 'crusty circles', the pruritus associated with these lesions, and the visible presence of epithelial collarettes and hyper-pigmented macules. Acetate tape strip cytology, taken from alopecic areas, shows only an occasional *Malassezia*. Low numbers of *Malassezia* are considered to be part of the normal skin microflora.

A *wet paper test* does not show any flea dirt. This is a quick and inexpensive test. A positive result is useful, especially for demonstrating tangible evidence of fleas to an owner. A negative result, as in this case, does not rule out the presence of fleas. Flea dirt is water soluble so swimming, or a recent bath, will affect the interpretation of the test. Alopecia over the caudal dorsum and tail base is commonly associated with flea bite hypersensitivity.

Deep skin scrapes. No *Demodex* mites are found. The alopecia associated with demodicosis is often first seen on the face and feet. This dog has a history of initial hair loss on the muzzle, but the feet are unaffected.

Fungal culture. Hair plucks, from the edges of the hypotrichotic areas, are sent to the laboratory for fungal culture. No dermatophytes are grown. Dermatophytosis is most often a non-pruritic condition in the dog. However, some less host-adapted species of dermatophyte can cause active folliculitis and pruritus. The owner, and the other two dogs, have no apparent skin lesions but this does not rule out the condition. The author has seen cases of dermatophytosis in which only one animal in a group has active infection and overt clinical signs.

A *urine cortisol: creatinine ratio* is 6.3×10^6, a normal ratio is $<30 \times 10^6$. This test has a high sensitivity, thus a result within the normal range effectively rules out a diagnosis of hyperadrenocorticism.

Haematology shows a low red blood cell count $4.42 \times 10^{12} \, l^{-1}$ ($5.5–8.5 \times 10^{12} \, l^{-1}$).

Serum biochemistry shows a raised alkaline phosphatase (ALP) $161 \, iu \, l^{-1}$ ($14–105 \, iu \, l^{-1}$), raised alanine aminotransferase (ALT) $377 \, iu \, l^{-1}$ ($13–88 \, iu \, l^{-1}$) and raised gamma-glutamyltransferase (GGT) $28.3 \, iu \, l^{-1}$ ($0–10 \, iu \, l^{-1}$).

The total T4 is low $8.5 \, nmol \, l^{-1}$ ($15–50 \, nmol \, l^{-1}$), and the thyroid stimulating hormone (TSH) value is elevated $1.56 \, ng \, ml^{-1}$ ($0.0–0.6 \, ng \, ml^{-1}$). The TSH assay result can also be elevated in normal dogs and those with concurrent illness. TSH can have a value within the normal range in hypothyroid dogs, making it best interpreted in combination with total T4.

Diagnosis

Hypothyroidism. The diagnosis is made by finding a combination of low total T4 (or free T4 by equilibrium dialysis) and elevated TSH in a dog with compatible clinical signs. There is also a secondary bacterial superficial pyoderma.

Treatment

Oral supplementation is started with sodium levothyroxine 600 µg, given every 12 hours. The total T4 result, *after 2 months on supplementation*, is $50.6 \, nmol \, l^{-1}$ ($15–50 \, nmol \, l^{-1}$). The blood sample is taken 4–6 hours after a dose of levothyroxine. Clinical evaluation of the patient is always more important than chasing numbers but this is a good result. It is at the top end of the normal range, and not exceeding $70 \, nmol \, l^{-1}$.

The owner comments that the dog is much more physically active and mentally alert. They had not noticed the previous lethargy and dullness, as this had developed in a slowly progressive fashion over a period of several months. The appearance of the skin and coat is largely unchanged, but there have been no further episodes of bacterial superficial pyoderma and the dog is not pruritic.

After 4 months of supplementation the total T4 result, taken 4–6 hours post pill, is $47.3 \, nmol \, l^{-1}$ ($15–50 \, nmol \, l^{-1}$). There is good early hair regrowth at the previously alopecic areas.

The dog achieved good hair regrowth, and a normal coat appearance, after 6–7 months of thyroxine supplementation.

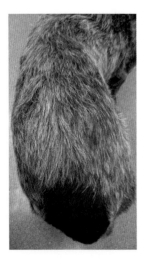

Figure 2.5 Shows the caudal dorsum from above. New hair has regrown to completely fill the previously alopecic and hypotrichotic areas. The new hair has more lustre and a more robust texture.

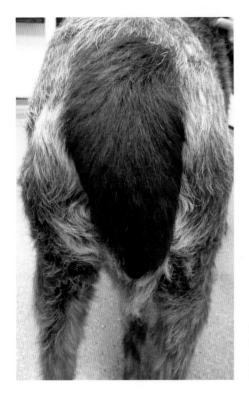

Figure 2.6 Shows the tail and rump from behind. The new hairs in the brown areas are darker coloured and more lustrous than the previous dull, red/brown hairs. Both post treatment photographs are taken after 12 months of supplementation with L-thyroxine.

Prognosis

The dog has a good response to treatment, so the prognosis is good for successful ongoing management with oral supplementation.

Discussion

Clinical signs started at just under 3 years of age in this case. Primary hypothyroidism is most commonly a disease of middle age, but cases with a younger onset are not uncommon. The waxing and waning pruritus seen in this Spinone was due to recurrent superficial pyoderma. There was no underlying pruritic skin condition and the bacterial skin infections stopped when the dog became euthyroid.

Approximately 30% of hypothyroid dogs, as in this case, have a low grade normochromic non-regenerative anaemia. A reduced production of red blood cells occurs in response to the reduced metabolic rate of the hypothyroid individual. The mildly elevated serum biochemistry values are non-specific and can be seen with hypothyroidism.

Total T4 concentrations can be difficult to interpret. They are influenced by a range of non-thyroid factors such as concurrent illness, breed, age and medication. Concurrent illness tends to reduce total T4 levels, but to an unpredictable degree. Sight hounds, such as Greyhounds and Salukis, have 'normal for breed' T4 levels that are low in comparison to other breeds. Young growing dogs have a higher set point for their metabolic rate and a corresponding higher T4 level, while in older dogs the T4 levels and metabolic rates tend to be lower. A variety of medications need to be considered when interpreting thyroid results; for example, total T4 can be reduced by the concurrent administration of carprofen, glucocorticoids, phenobarbitone or sulfonamide antibiotics.

A total T4 value in the normal range usually rules out a diagnosis of hypothyroidism. When values are low it is helpful to look at the concurrent TSH value. Approximately 65% of hypothyroid dogs will have an elevated TSH value.

Thyroid hormone is required to move the hair follicle cycle into an actively growing (anagen) phase. Hypothyroid dogs have a relatively high proportion of hairs arrested at the telogen phase. Retained hairs are old and may appear dull, and bleached in colour. The resting hairs are eventually shed and are not replaced, leading to alopecia. The pattern of hair loss varies but typically includes an inverted V shape on the dorsal rostral muzzle, bilaterally symmetrical flank alopecia, and/or an alopecic 'rat' tail. None of these hair loss patterns are pathognomic for hypothyroidism. A few breeds, such as the Irish Setter, can have densely packed retained hairs giving a 'carpet coat' appearance.

Further reading

Daminet, S. and Ferguson, D. (2003). Influence of drugs on thyroid function in dogs. *Journal of Veterinary Internal Medicine* 17: 463–472.

Graham, P.A., Refsal, K.R., and Nachreiner, R.F. (2007). Etiopathologic findings of canine hypothyroidism. *Veterinary Clinics of North America Small Animal Practice* 37: 617–631.

Smiley, L.E. and Peterson, M.E. (1993). Evaluation of a urine cortisol: creatinine ratio as a screening test for hyperadrenocorticism in dogs. *Journal of Veterinary Internal Medicine* 7: 163–168.

History

A 7 year-old female entire domestic short-haired cat is presented because of hair loss. Thinning of the hair coat was noticed on the caudal hind limbs, starting 6 weeks ago, and has progressed dorsally and cranially since that time. The owners have not seen the cat display any excessive self-grooming behaviour, but they have seen fur balls regurgitated on an almost daily basis. There is another cat in the household, which has no clinical signs of skin disease. Both cats have an indoor and outdoor lifestyle, with the unrestricted use of a cat flap. Both cats have regular routine vaccinations and intermittent flea and anthelmintic treatment.

Questions

1. Describe the abnormalities and pertinent normal features in Figures 3.1–3.3.
2. What differential diagnoses should be considered for this presentation?
3. What tests could you perform to make the diagnosis?

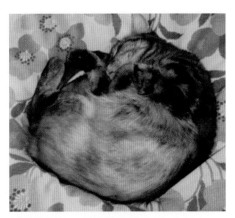

Figure 3.1

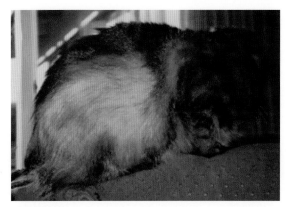

Figure 3.2

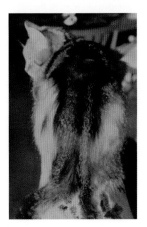

Figure 3.3

Small Animal Dermatology: What's Your Diagnosis? First Edition. Jane Coatesworth.
© 2019 John Wiley & Sons, Inc. Published 2019 by John Wiley & Sons, Inc.

Answers

1. What the figures show

Figure 3.1 shows the cat curled up asleep. There is a large area of partial alopecia over the left flank and the left proximal hind limb.

Figure 3.2 shows the right side of the body. There is a large patch of alopecia extending from the mid-thorax to the perineum, and from the sub-lumbar fossa to the mid-thigh. The tail base and the proximomedial hind limbs are also alopecic.

Figure 3.3 shows the cat from behind. There is bilateral symmetry of the flank alopecia. The hair coat over the tail and dorsal mid-line have a normal appearance.

2. Differential diagnoses

Given the appearance of the skin lesions the following conditions should be considered:

Causes of alopecia due to excessive self-grooming:

- Flea bite hypersensitivity
- Cutaneous adverse food reaction
- Atopic dermatitis
- Psychogenic alopecia
- Demodicosis (*Demodex gatoi*)

Causes of alopecia due to excessive hair shedding:

- Dermatophytosis
- Demodicosis (*Demodex cati*)
- Bacterial folliculitis
- Hyperadrenocorticism
- Diabetes mellitus
- Telogen defluxion

3. Appropriate diagnostic tests

General physical examination is unremarkable. The cat is bright and well.

Trichogram. Clumps of hair are plucked from the margin of the alopecic areas. The hairs are difficult to epilate, suggesting that the hair coat is not in telogen arrest. There are numerous fractured hair shafts, and a mixture of anagen and telogen bulbs. No fungal elements or *Demodex* mites are seen. The damage to the hair shafts is likely to be self-inflicted by vigorous over-grooming, albeit done in private. The regular production of fur balls supports this suspicion. A trichogram is a useful, fast and inexpensive test to differentiate alopecia due to excessive grooming (difficult epilation and broken shafts) from alopecia due to excessive shedding (easily epilated telogen hairs and intact hair tips).

Wet paper testing shows a few flea dirts, confirming the recent presence of fleas on the cat. Flea dirt is water soluble, so it may be totally removed from the coat of a pruritic cat that is washing itself excessively, even if fleas are present in high numbers. The absence of flea dirts does not indicate that fleas are not present.

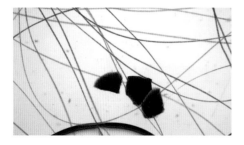

Figure 3.4 Shows part of a coat brushing mounted in liquid paraffin under a glass cover slip. There is a fragmented flea dirt among several loose hairs.

Superficial and deep skin scrapes do not reveal any *Demodex* mites. The short-bodied *D. gatoi* mites live in the stratum corneum and are sampled by acetate tape strips or superficial skin scrapes. *D. cati* mites, in comparison, live down the hair follicles and are sampled by deeper skin scrapes to the point of capillary oozing. Increased *D. cati* numbers are usually seen in association with immunosuppression. *D. gatoi* can cause marked pruritus and, unlike *D. cati*, is considered to be contagious between cats. In this case, the other cat in the household was unaffected by skin disease.

Fungal culture was established using hairs plucked from the margins of the alopecic areas. A Wood's lamp could be used to look for fluorescence in infected hairs. Dermatophytosis usually causes non pruritic alopecia in the cat, but can occasionally be pruritic and lead to alopecia through self-trauma. The bilaterally symmetrical pattern would be unusual, but dermatophytosis does have a highly pleomorphic clinical presentation.

Diagnosis

Flea bite hypersensitivity is the most likely diagnosis. Other causes of alopecia due to excessive grooming, apart from *D. gatoi*, cannot be ruled out at this stage. Performing a robust food trial needs commitment and perseverance from an owner, and atopic dermatitis is a diagnosis made by exclusion. A pragmatic approach is to assess the response to robust flea control before undertaking a food trial.

Treatment

Many commercial products are available for flea control. The aim of treatment is to reduce the number of flea bites to a low enough level, such that the hypersensitivity reaction is not triggered. Some cats may also need short-term symptomatic antipruritic therapy to improve their welfare. Considerations in this case are to treat the indoor environment, to kill adult fleas seeking a blood meal on both cats and to treat the potential outdoor environments that the cats visit and where fleas may be breeding.

Indoor environmental control needs an investment of time, energy and money to be effective. This can be undertaken by the pet owner or by a professional pest controller. Environmental control is an important aspect of overall treatment, as the majority of the flea lifecycle is harboured in the environment. The persistence of eggs, larvae and pupae acts as a reservoir for infestation with adult fleas. Pupae, in their protective cocoons, are difficult to kill and can persist for many months. Vacuum cleaning of the floor and soft furnishings is a helpful initial stage. Vacuum cleaning removes the organic debris and flea dirt on which the flea larvae feed and introduces vibration that stimulates adult fleas to emerge from their cocoons. Vacuum cleaned areas should include favourite cat resting places, under the seat cushions of furniture and anywhere dark at floor level, for example underneath the sofa. The floor area of the house and any soft furnishings where the cats rest should be sprayed with an environmental spray. Sprays usually contain a rapid knock-down component such as permethrin and a persistent insect growth regulator such as pyriproxyfen or fenoxycarb.

The choice of *adulticide treatment* is often limited by the practicalities of administration. The owner felt unable to give any oral products and did not want the cat to wear a collar. Spot-on treatments were a practical choice in this case. A spot-on product with systemic absorption and redistribution of the active ingredient is helpful in cats with vigorous and extensive over-grooming. It is important to treat all of the in contact animals.

Environmental control outside of the house is particularly difficult and can be addressed by spot-on products containing methoprene or imidocloprid. These are shed with skin scale into the environment of a resting cat and will have some impact on the lifecycle. Known resting places outside of the house should be specifically targeted, but great care should be taken with environmental sprays. Permethrin is highly toxic to beneficial insect life, such as honeybees and hover flies, and is toxic to fish and aquatic invertebrates if it gets into water courses. Flea eggs are killed by a couple of days of sub-zero temperatures, but may survive outdoors in temperature protected niches.

Symptomatic treatment for itch and inflammation is often helpful in the short-term management of flea bite hypersensitivity. Hydrocortisone aceponate spray has been shown to improve both lesion scores and the degree of itch in cats with presumed allergy. Most of the clinical improvement was seen in the first 14 days of treatment. This product is not licensed for use in the cat. A short course of oral prednisolone can also be effective. This cat was not given any symptomatic treatment for itch and inflammation, due to poor compliance with oral medication and owner perception that the application of a spray formulation would be difficult to achieve.

Re-inspections and final outcome

No growth occurs on the fungal culture after 2 weeks of incubation.

One month later the hair coat is re-growing. The owner reports a reduced frequency of hair balls. There is a small amount of flea dirt on a wet paper test.

After a further month, the owner reports the return of a full hair coat.

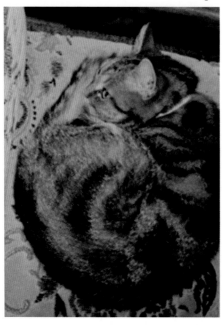

Figure 3.5 Shows the cat 2 months after initial presentation. There is full regrowth of the hair coat at the previously alopecic areas.

Seven months later, the cat is seen again with symmetrical alopecia down the caudal hind limbs and over the flanks. A wet paper test shows a moderate amount of flea dirt, and a trichogram shows barbered hairs. The owner had stopped using flea control on the other cat in the household after a 6-month period. The need for ongoing treatment for both of the cats is explained again to the owner.

Three weeks later there was some hair regrowth and an occasional flea dirt on wet paper test.

A final diagnosis of flea bite hypersensitivity was made based on the demonstration of flea dirt concurrent with clinical signs, the reduction of flea dirt and clinical signs following flea control measures and the recurrence of clinical signs when flea control was inadequate.

Prognosis

The prognosis is good, if fleas can be effectively controlled on an ongoing basis.

Discussion

Flea bite hypersensitivity is a common condition in the cat. Clinical signs vary from self-induced alopecia in the inguinal or lumbosacral area, to miliary crusting dermatitis around the neck and dorsum and eosinophilic plaques, ulcers or granulomas. None of these clinical presentations are unique for flea bite hypersensitivity and, as with many dermatological patterns, other differential diagnoses need to be considered.

The recurrence of clinical signs, when the other cat in the household had not been treated for 2 months, suggests that the untreated cat and the environment was supporting a significant flea population. These fleas were probably biting the hypersensitive cat enough to trigger clinical signs, despite ongoing treatment of that individual. This case demonstrates that the level of environmental challenge is an important factor for the protection of hypersensitive individuals, as well as their regular individual treatment. It is not uncommon for owners to concentrate their treatment efforts exclusively onto the affected animal and to undertreat the other pets within a multi-pet household. The other cat in this household shared the same environment but showed no clinical signs.

Flea control needs to be sustained in the long term, in the environment of a hypersensitive pet. Owners need information about the flea lifecycle and suitable insecticidal products. They also need realistic expectations of time scales, cost and the amount of work required to control and prevent infestations. Significant flea infestations are likely to take at least 3 months to bring under control. The degree of necessary flea control may vary between cases, as the threshold of sensitivity is likely to vary between individuals and may vary in affected individuals over their lifetime.

Further reading

Carlotti, D. and Jacobs, D. (2000). Therapy, control and prevention of flea allergy dermatitis in dogs and cats. *Veterinary Dermatology* 11: 83–98.

Schmidt, V., Buckley, L.M., McEwan, N.A. et al. (2012). Efficacy of a 0.584% hydrocortisone aceponate spray in presumed feline allergic dermatitis: an open label pilot study. *Veterinary Dermatology* 23: 11–16.

History

A 5 year-old male neutered Old English Sheepdog is presented with an 8-month history of pruritus. The dog has been with the owners since a puppy, and is regularly dewormed and vaccinated. The other dog in the household has crusted papules on the abdomen and flanks, and is moderately pruritic. Both dogs receive topical fipronil, given every 5 months, for flea control. The owners initially noticed scratching at one elbow and at the top of the head. The extent and severity of the skin signs, and the degree of pruritus, have steadily progressed. The owners do not have any skin lesions or pruritus. There is no response to an 8-week food trial with a commercial novel protein diet, to four months of essential fatty acid supplementation or to frequent bathing with a chlorhexidine based shampoo. There are transient reductions in pruritus after injections of dexamethasone and a sustained reduction in pruritus on twice daily oclacitinib. Reducing the dose of oclacitinib to once daily results in the pruritus returning to a high level. The owners give the itch score as 9/10, with almost constant scratching, rubbing and biting over the entire body, including during the night. An Elizabethan collar is placed on the dog when he is alone, to prevent self-excoriation of the head and ears and biting at the body. The dog has become depressed in demeanour over the past few weeks. He has a poor appetite and has lost a little weight.

Questions

1. Describe the abnormalities and pertinent normal features in Figures 4.1–4.4.
2. What differential diagnoses should be considered for this presentation?
3. What tests could you perform to make the diagnosis?

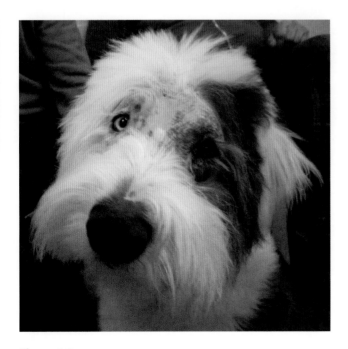

Figure 4.1

Small Animal Dermatology: What's Your Diagnosis? First Edition. Jane Coatesworth.
© 2019 John Wiley & Sons, Inc. Published 2019 by John Wiley & Sons, Inc.

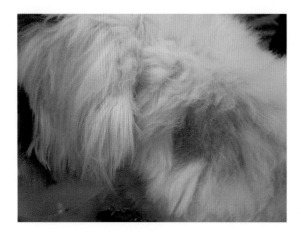

Figure 4.2

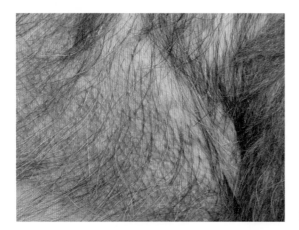

Figure 4.3

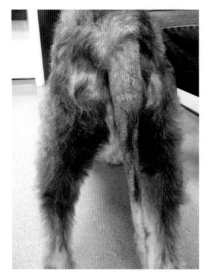

Figure 4.4

Answers

1. **What the figures show**

    Figure 4.1 shows the dog's face. There is an extensive area of total alopecia around and between the eyes. There is an accumulation of thick yellow crust at the top and midline of the alopecic area. The exposed skin is erythematous.

    Figure 4.2 shows the left lateral neck and pinna. There is marked generalised erythema. The hair coat over the caudal aspect of the pinna is very thin. There is an approximately 10 cm diameter alopecic patch on the lateral neck and some excoriations.

    Figure 4.3 shows the glabrous area behind the right elbow. There are numerous, often confluent erythematous papules.

    Figure 4.4 shows the rear view of the dog. There is marked generalised erythema of the skin and multifocal aggregates of thick yellow crust and scale. The tail is almost totally alopecic and there are large patches of alopecia over the caudal pelvis, with an area of excoriation on the left side. The alopecic point of hock is just visible on the right side.

2. **Differential diagnoses**

    Given the appearance of the skin lesions the following conditions should be considered:

    • Sarcoptic mange

3. **Appropriate diagnostic tests**

    Superficial skin scrapings. Two adult mites are found, after multiple skin scrapings from a variety of body sites including the caudal pinna.

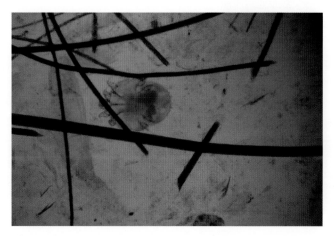

Figure 4.5 Shows detail from a skin scraping, mounted in liquid paraffin and examined under the microscope, with the ×10 lens. There is an eight legged adult *Sarcoptes* mite with head to the left, among the fragments of hair shaft. *Sarcoptes* mites have short legs and the two hind pairs do not extend beyond the outline of the body. The two pairs of front legs have long unjointed stalks with terminal suckers.

    A *pinnal scratch reflex* is readily elicited. This test is performed by folding the pinna, rubbing the two sections of pinna together and watching for the hind leg on the same side to perform a scratching motion. The test is not entirely specific for *Sarcoptes* infestation, but a positive response increases the diagnostic suspicion.

Diagnosis

Sarcoptic mange.

Treatment

Oral sarolaner at 2–4 mg kg^{-1} is given to both dogs and repeated after 1 month.

Oral prednisolone is given at 1 mg kg^{-1} once daily for 5 days, then at 0.5 mg kg^{-1} once daily for 5 days, then at 0.5 mg kg^{-1} every other day for 20 days. The prednisolone is given in the morning with food.

The house and car are sprayed with a permethrin based acaricidal spray, to kill any mites surviving in the environment.

Contact with other dogs is avoided apart from the second dog in the household, which is likely to be affected already. The zoonotic potential is discussed with the owners.

The dog is bathed twice weekly with an aloe and oatmeal emollient shampoo.

After 1 month of treatment the dog is much brighter in demeanour and has a good appetite. The body weight has increased to normal and stabilised. The level of pruritus has reduced to 6/10, with intermittent scratching and rubbing at the head and legs. The previously excoriated and eroded areas have healed and there is early hair regrowth at previously alopecic areas. Oral prednisolone is continued and bathing reduced to weekly.

After a further month of treatment the itch score has reduced to 3/10. Prednisolone and bathing are discontinued. There is further good quality hair regrowth.

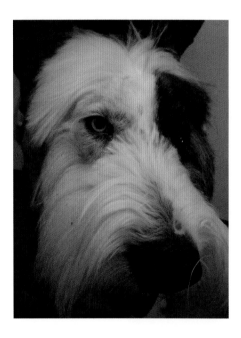

Figure 4.6 Shows the dog's head after 2 months of treatment. There is good quality hair regrowth at the previously alopecic area, around and between the eyes. The thick crust has resolved and the dog has a more relaxed and alert appearance.

The owners report that it took a further 2 months for the level of pruritus to return to normal.

Prognosis

The prognosis is excellent, as infestation with *Sarcoptes* is a curable condition.

Discussion

A lack of demonstrable mites, eggs or faecal pellets, on skin scraping does not exclude a diagnosis of sarcoptic mange. An enzyme-linked immunosorbent assay (ELISA) test, which measures immunoglobulin G (IgG) to *Sarcoptes* antigens, is useful when no mites are found. This serology test has a high sensitivity and specificity. False negatives can occur in the first month of infestation as not enough IgG may have been generated to flag up the presence of mites. False positives can occur if the dog is allergic to house dust mites (*Dermatophagoides*) and is mounting high levels of IgG to shared antigens. Interestingly, antibody cross reactivity does not seem to be an issue with ectoparasite infestations involving fleas, *Otodectes* or *Cheyletiella*. A false positive reaction could also occur when a previous *Sarcoptes* infestation has clinically resolved. A high *Sarcoptes* titre, post exposure, persists for a variable amount of time but is likely to have returned to normal after six months. This variability in persistence may relate to differing rates of antigen clearance from the body, as antigen is still physically present after the mites have been killed.

The isoxazolines, including sarolaner, lotilaner, fluralaner and afoxolaner, work by blocking the GABA and glutamate gated chlorine channels in the central nervous system of both insects and mites. While the isoxazoline family has shown clinical efficacy against *Sarcoptes*, only sarolaner is currently licensed in the United Kingdom for the treatment of sarcoptic mange.

Further reading

Bornstein, S. and Zacrisson, G. (1993). Humoral antibody response to experimental *Sarcoptes scabiei* var. *vulpes* infection in the dog. *Veterinary Dermatology* 4: 107–110.

Mueller, R., Bettenay, S.V., and Shipstone, M. (2001). Value of the pinnal-pedal scratch reflex in the diagnosis of canine scabies. *Veterinary Record* 148: 621–623.

History

A 13 year-old male neutered domestic short-haired cat is presented because of recent patchy hair loss. The owners have noticed progressive weight loss, starting 3–4 months ago. Biting of the paws and resentment of paw handling started shortly after the weight loss. A patch of alopecia is first noticed at the left axilla 3 weeks ago. The extent of the alopecia progresses rapidly to include the medial aspects of all four limbs and the entire ventrum. The cat has been drinking more over the past 2 weeks. More recently the owners have noticed a degree of unsteadiness on the hind limbs, and increased washing of the legs and paws.

Questions

1. Describe the abnormalities and pertinent normal features in Figures 5.1–5.5.
2. What differential diagnoses should be considered for this presentation?
3. What tests could you perform to make the diagnosis?

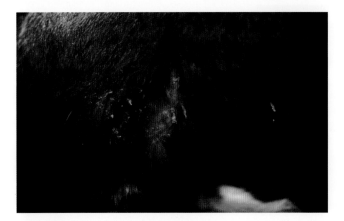

Figure 5.1

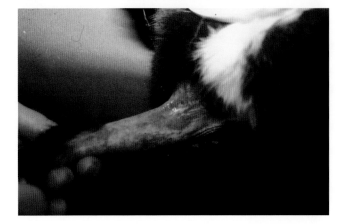

Figure 5.2

Small Animal Dermatology: What's Your Diagnosis? First Edition. Jane Coatesworth.
© 2019 John Wiley & Sons, Inc. Published 2019 by John Wiley & Sons, Inc.

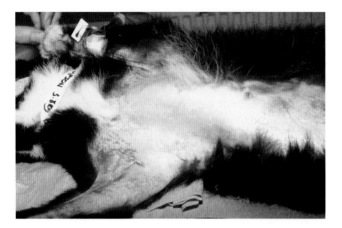

Figure 5.3

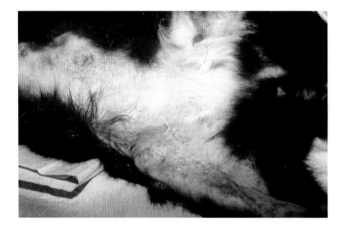

Figure 5.4

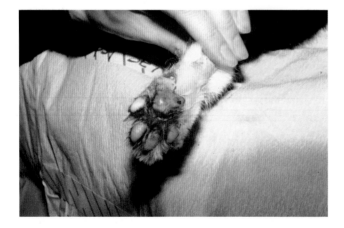

Figure 5.5

Answers

1. What the figures show

Figure 5.1 shows the right lateral hind limb. The hair coat contains excess scale, is easily epilated and is being shed in tufts. The remaining hair coat is dull and dry.

Figure 5.2 shows the right medial forelimb. There is total alopecia from the axilla to the carpus. The exposed skin has a glistening and smooth appearance.

Figure 5.3 shows the ventral chest and medial forelimbs. There is extensive bilaterally symmetrical alopecia. Sutures are visible at the skin biopsy site in the right axilla.

Figure 5.4 shows the ventral abdomen, groin and medial right hind limb. There is extensive alopecia and the skin has a smooth appearance. Skin biopsies have been taken from the right groin and left medial thigh.

Figure 5.5 shows the left hind paw. The interdigital spaces contain a sticky, matted, black material. The paw pads have a smooth and shiny surface. All of the feet have a similar appearance. The skin around the nailbeds is alopecic and erythematous.

2. Differential diagnoses

Given the appearance of the skin lesions the following conditions should be considered:

- Paraneoplastic alopecia. This older cat, with rapidly progressive symmetrical ventral alopecia, combined with weight loss, has a typical history and clinical appearance of feline paraneoplastic alopecia.
- Hyperadrenocorticism. Approximately half of cases of feline hyperadrenocorticism show cutaneous signs. Signs are very variable and include bilaterally symmetrical alopecia, making hyperadrenocorticism a differential diagnosis here. This cat, in common with most feline hyperadrenocorticism cases, also has increased thirst and is in the older age bracket. Approximately 90% of cats with hyperadrenocorticism are insulin resistant and show consequent lethargy, polyphagia, polydypsia and polyuria. They may show weight loss or weight gain. The skin in this case is thin, but does not show the skin fragility often associated with hyperadrenocorticism. The striking smooth shiny appearance of the skin and the ventral bilaterally symmetrical alopecia seen in this case are not typical of hyperadrenocorticism.
- Hyperthyroidism is common in older cats and may present with weight loss, increased thirst, an unkempt appearance and over-grooming behaviour. However, the distinctive ventral pattern of symmetrical alopecia and the smooth shiny skin are not suggestive of hyperthyroidism. This cat has a reduced appetite and is lethargic while hyperthyroid cats typically, but not exclusively, eat increased amounts of food and have increased activity levels due to a raised metabolic rate.

3. Appropriate diagnostic tests

Physical examination. The cat is lethargic and inactive. At 3.8 kg the cat is underweight, compared to a usual recorded body weight of 4.9 kg. There are increased lung sounds on thoracic auscultation.

Haematology and serum biochemistry, including blood glucose, are unremarkable. Haematology and biochemistry profiles have been found to be unremarkable, or to show only slight non-specific changes, in cases of paraneoplastic alopecia.

Thoracic and abdominal radiographs. The thoracic radiographs show a bronchial and interstitial pattern consistent with advanced age. No abnormalities are detected on the abdominal images.

Cytology of the black interdigital material shows high numbers of *Malassezia* yeasts.

Full thickness *skin biopsies* are taken from the centre of areas of alopecic skin. Histopathology shows hyperplastic perivascular dermatitis and deep follicular atrophy, suggestive of paraneoplastic alopecia. Histopathology of paraneoplastic alopecia typically shows changes that include absence of the stratum corneum, telogen arrest, follicular miniaturisation and moderate to severe acanthosis. The distinctive shiny appearance of the alopecic skin is thought to be associated with the absence of stratum corneum.

Diagnosis and prognosis

Feline paraneoplastic alopecia. The owner was offered an exploratory laparotomy to confirm the diagnosis of an underlying neoplastic disease. Exploratory laparotomy can also allow a search for the presence of visible metastases, and/or the removal of the primary tumour.

Prognosis

The cat has a very poor prognosis. Feline paraneoplastic alopecia is reversible if the underlying cause can be identified and successfully treated. However, the types of neoplasia that underlie this paraneoplastic syndrome generally carry a poor prognosis. The clinical signs in this case have been present for several months, making it very likely that metastasis has already occurred.

Final outcome

The owners opt for euthanasia.

Post mortem examination shows a firm white mass at the junction of the pancreatic lobes, with a diameter of 4 mm. The liver and lung lobes contain multiple firm white masses of 1–3 mm diameter. Histopathology reveals a pancreatic acinar cell carcinoma with metastases to the liver, lymph nodes and lungs.

Discussion

The underlying neoplasia in this case is a pancreatic carcinoma. There are approximately 20 cases of feline paraneoplastic alopecia reported in the literature. The majority have pancreatic neoplasia, while others have primary tumours in the bile duct or liver. Feline paraneoplastic alopecia is a rare disease but the distinctive clinical signs are a readily recognised cutaneous marker of internal malignancy. The disease is typically seen in older cats and weight loss is a common feature. The systemic clinical signs reflect the underlying neoplasia and can include poor appetite, lethargy, vomiting and diarrhoea.

Radiography was unhelpful in this case for visualising the primary and secondary tumours. The multiple pulmonary lesions were not evident on thoracic radiography. They were found at post mortem examination to have a diameter of 1–3 mm. Non-mineralised soft tissue lesions of such small diameter do not register on radiographs. The primary tumour was not seen on the abdominal radiographs. There was poor contrast on the abdominal films as the cat had very little abdominal fat. Ultrasonography or magnetic resonance imaging would have been a more sensitive choice of imaging techniques to demonstrate the pancreatic primary, and the hepatic and pulmonary secondary lesions.

Most cases of feline paraneoplastic alopecia, as with this case, have metastases present at the time of diagnosis. Complete resolution of the cutaneous signs, following surgical removal of a pancreatic primary tumour, has been described in two cats. In both of these cases there were no apparent metastases seen at exploratory laparotomy. Histopathology of lymph nodes and liver biopsies showed no metastases when taken at the time of surgery in one case, but the alopecia recurred four months after surgery. The cat was subsequently euthanised and metastases were found on post mortem examination.

Uncomplicated feline paraneoplastic alopecia is a non-pruritic condition but, in common with many skin disorders, it can be complicated by secondary microbial infections and/or overgrowths. *Malassezia* interdigital dermatitis is a feature of this case and may have been the cause of the pedal discomfort and paw biting. Another case of feline paraneoplastic alopecia with secondary *Malassezia*-associated dermatitis showed lower limb pruritus as a prominent clinical sign. The pruritus in that case resolved within a few days of treatment with 5 mg kg^{-1} ketoconazole twice daily. Three other reported cases of paraneoplastic alopecia, with underlying pancreatic carcinoma, had concurrent *Malassezia* dermatitis. Two of these were pruritic.

Further reading

Brooks, D.G., Campbell, K.L., Dennis, J.S. et al. (1994). Pancreatic paraneoplastic alopecia in three cats. *Journal of the American Animal Hospital Association* 30: 557–563.

Caporali, C. (2016). Two cases of feline paraneoplastic alopecia associated with a neuroendocrine pancreatic neoplasia and a hepatosplenic plasma cell tumour. *Veterinary Dermatology* 27: 508–512.

Godfrey, D.R. (1998). A case of feline paraneoplastic alopecia with secondary *Malassezia*-associated dermatitis. *Journal of Small Animal Practice* 39: 394–396.

Pascal-Tenorio, A., Olivry, T., Gross, T.L. et al. (1997). Paraneoplastic alopecia associated with internal malignancies in the cat. *Veterinary Dermatology* 8: 47–52.

Tasker, S., Griffon, D.J., Nuttall, T.J. et al. (1999). Resolution of paraneoplastic alopecia following surgical removal of a pancreatic carcinoma in a cat. *Journal of Small Animal Practice* 40: 16–19.

History

A 4 year-old female entire Dobermann is presented with a history of thinning of the hair coat. The hair thinning was first seen over the trunk and neck area, and started at 6 months of age. The dog was diagnosed with and treated for juvenile onset generalised demodicosis and secondary bacterial superficial pyoderma at that time. The hair coat regrew on the neck, after treatment for the demodicosis, but did not fully regrow on the trunk. Since then occasional episodes of bacterial pyoderma have recurred, but no *Demodex* mites have been found associated with these recurrent episodes. The dog is mildly pruritic when pyoderma is present, but the pruritus resolves completely when the pyoderma is treated. The hair loss over the trunk has progressed very slowly over the years. In the past 6 months, the back of the head has also shown progressive hair loss. The dog is bright and active, with no systemic clinical signs or current pruritus. There are no other pets in the household and the dog is regularly vaccinated and dewormed.

Questions

1. Describe the abnormalities and pertinent normal features in Figures 6.1–6.3.
2. What differential diagnoses should be considered for this presentation?
3. What tests could you perform to make the diagnosis?

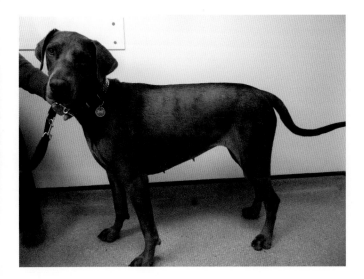

Figure 6.1

Small Animal Dermatology: What's Your Diagnosis? First Edition. Jane Coatesworth.
© 2019 John Wiley & Sons, Inc. Published 2019 by John Wiley & Sons, Inc.

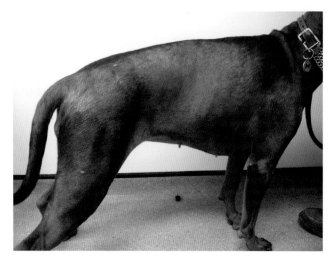

Figure 6.2

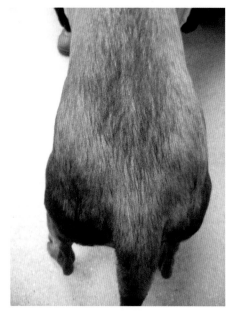

Figure 6.3

Answers

1. What the figures show

Figure 6.1 shows an extensive patch of alopecia over the lateral trunk and another over the rostral chest. The head and flank fold areas are hypotrichotic. The tan hair coat at the eyebrows, muzzle and distal limbs has a normal appearance.

Figure 6.2 shows that the pattern of hair loss is bilaterally symmetrical. The tan hair coat at the perineum and distal limbs has a normal appearance.

Figure 6.3 shows extensive hypotrichosis to alopecia over the dorsal trunk and tail base. The dorsal midline is relatively spared. The skin is dry and scaly.

2. Differential diagnoses

Given the appearance of the skin lesions the following conditions should be considered:

- Recurrent generalised demodicosis. The dog has a history of juvenile onset generalised demodicosis. A small proportion of these cases recur after successful initial treatment and need ongoing management.

- Colour dilution alopecia. The dog has a blue coat colour. This, along with fawn, is one of the dilute colours for the breed and makes it at risk of developing colour dilution alopecia (CDA).
- Dermatophytosis can cause generalised alopecia with no associated pruritus.
- Endocrinopathies, for example hypothyroidism, hyperadrenocorticism. These are unlikely as the dog has an early age of onset and has no compatible clinical signs other than recurrent pyoderma and symmetrical alopecia.

3. **Appropriate diagnostic tests**

Physical examination. General physical examination is unremarkable, and there is no evidence of bacterial pyoderma. Running a hand over the skin reveals a number of short broken hairs with a 'stubble' texture.

Hair plucks and deep skin scrapes show no *Demodex* mites. Hair plucks are taken first, as these are quick and non-traumatic for the dog. When these show no mites, deep skin scrapes are taken to rule out demodicosis. Hair plucks show hair shafts containing clumps of large and irregular melanin aggregates. Some of the hair shafts are fractured.

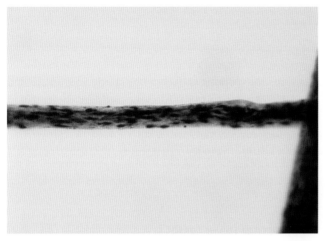

Figure 6.4 Shows a plucked hair from the dog. There is abnormal melanin clumping within the hair shaft. The profile of the hair is undulating and irregular in comparison to the more linear margins seen in a normal dog.

Dermatophyte culture of the hair coat, sampled with a McKenzie brush technique, shows no dermatophyte growth.

Haematology and serum biochemistry are unremarkable, giving useful information prior to anaesthesia.

Total T4 and thyroid stimulating hormone (TSH) assay are unremarkable, ruling out hypothyroidism.

Urine cortisol: creatinine ratio is normal, ruling out hyperadrenocorticism.

Skin biopsies. Three 8 mm full-thickness punch biopsies are taken under general anaesthetic. As with most alopecic conditions, it is helpful to take the biopsies from the most obviously alopecic areas. Histopathology shows prominent clumps of pigment both surrounding and throughout the length of the hair follicles and inside the hair shafts. The hair follicles have bizarre distorted shapes and show a mixture of anagen and telogen phase activity. There will be abnormal clumping of melanin in the follicles and hair shafts of dilute coloured dogs that are not affected by CDA. Individuals with CDA have a greater degree of melanin aggregation, and have numerous dysplastic hair follicles.

Diagnosis

CDA, sometimes known as colour mutant alopecia.

Treatment

CDA is a largely cosmetic disease in an otherwise healthy dog. The sparse hair coat leaves the skin exposed to potential ultraviolet damage and the abnormal hair follicles are prone to repeated bacterial infections.

A topical emollient, containing a high sun protection factor sunscreen, should be used on the alopecic areas during the summer months. Sunscreen products either reflect or absorb ultraviolet light, or may have both actions. A well-fitting coat, made of a lightweight fabric that blocks ultraviolet light, can be used in the summer months but any skin abrasion is likely to hasten local hair loss.

Regular antimicrobial bathing, to reduce bacterial overpopulation on the skin. Bathing is followed by a conditioner to increase the flexibility and resilience of the remaining hair coat, and to maintain skin hydration. Vigorous rubbing of the hair coat is best avoided, as it can result in fracture of the brittle hairs. A stroking motion, in the direction of the hair coat, can be used while bathing, rinsing and applying conditioner. This approach is also helpful when bathing dogs with sebaceous adenitis.

The owners are keen to try additional therapy. Melatonin 3 mg is given every 8 hours for 6 weeks then, when there is no response, increased to 8 mg every 8 hours for 6 weeks. The owners are advised that there is only anecdotal evidence for this treatment and that it is unlikely to be effective. Melatonin is maintained for 1 year, with little appreciable change in the hair coat.

Prognosis

The prognosis is good, with ongoing care of the skin. The alopecia is likely to be slowly progressive and ultimately irreversible, but the condition is largely of cosmetic concern. Alopecic areas are vulnerable to increased levels of ultraviolet irradiation and consequent related damage. The presence of fractured hairs in this dog and the anagen bulbs seen on histopathology suggest that there is still capacity to regrow some hair coat. CDA tends to have a steady progression from early broken hairs that regrow, through to complete alopecia without hair regrowth.

Discussion

A dilute coat colour is a genetic modification of the normal colour for the breed. The majority of Dobermann Pinschers have a black coat with tan (also called rust) coloured markings. The black colour, in the presence of two copies of the dilution allele (dd), is diluted to various shades of blue. The tan markings are not diluted. The melanin granules within individual hairs are arranged abnormally in dogs with dilute coat colours and very abnormally in individuals with CDA. The inherent pigment colour (eumelanin) is the same in black and dilute black (i.e. blue) dogs. It is the distribution of the pigment that causes the apparent colour variation. Dilute hairs do not contain a reduced amount of pigment, but have pigment stored differently within the hairs. The colour referred to as brown in the UK, or red in the USA, is a recognised but less prevalent coat colour in the Dobermann. Brown/red dilutes to fawn. Dogs with blue or fawn coats are at risk of CDA. Although a single recessive gene is responsible for dilution of the coat colour, not all dogs with dilute colouring develop CDA. The additional factors needed to develop the disease are not yet fully understood. The dog in this case has a mid-blue hair coat and has moderate disease. Within the spectrum of a blue coat the lighter coloured individuals are typically more severely affected with CDA than darker coloured dogs and show hair loss at an earlier age.

This dog has a history of recurrent bacterial skin infections over the dorsum. These were initially ascribed to the juvenile onset generalised demodicosis. The follicular inflammation in demodicosis is commonly complicated by bacterial infection. Recurrent episodes persisted, despite resolution of the demodicosis, and the hair coat over the trunk did not completely regrow. This suggests that signs of CDA started at 6–12 months of age in this dog. The onset of clinical signs is usually seen in young adults, before four years of age. CDA is recognised in a wide range of breeds, and crossbreeds, which show dilute coat colours. These include the Dachshund, Great Dane, Yorkshire Terrier, Whippet, Greyhound and Chihuahua.

Hair loss usually starts over the trunk, and progresses to involve other areas. Regions of hair coat with undiluted colour, such as the tan coated areas in this case, are not affected. Affected hairs are brittle and easily broken by abrasive grooming and bathing, and by abrasion from coats or harnesses. The rate and presence of hair regrowth diminishes with time, resulting in progressive hypotrichosis then alopecia. The coat often feels dry and brittle and there is secondary scaling of the exposed skin, as in this dog. Some dogs develop prominent comedones where the dysplastic hair follicles are filled with sebum and cellular debris.

Hairs from normal dogs, with non-dilute coat colours, have small and evenly distributed aggregates of melanin throughout the hair shafts. Hairs from dilute coloured dogs without CDA show larger and more unevenly distributed aggregates of melanin and those with CDA have more pronounced changes. The presence of very large melanin aggregates, associated with hair shaft fracture, is suggestive of CDA but skin biopsy is recommended to confirm the diagnosis.

There is no effective treatment for CDA, but the progression of clinical signs and the frequency of secondary infections can be reduced by appropriate management. The condition has an autosomal recessive inheritance pattern and affected individuals should not be used for breeding. There is a genetic test available to identify individuals carrying the dilute (D locus) gene, but only a proportion of dogs with a dilute coat colour will develop CDA. There is not yet a specific genetic test available for CDA.

Further reading

Miller, W.H. (1990). Colour dilution alopecia in Doberman Pinschers with blue or fawn coats: a study on the incidence and histopathology of this disorder. *Veterinary Dermatology* 1: 113–122.

Roperto, F. (1995). Colour dilution alopecia (CDA) in ten Yorkshire Terriers. *Veterinary Dermatology* 6: 171–178.

History

A 10 year-old female neutered Staffordshire Bull Terrier cross is presented with a 12-month history of progressive alopecia. The alopecia has progressed most rapidly in the past 6 months. Thirteen months ago, the dog was spayed and had a unilateral mammary strip for mammary adenoma. The left forelimb was amputated for osteosarcoma 1 year ago. The dog became pruritic 6 months ago and has received daily prednisolone since then (at a dose varying between 0.5 and 2 mg kg^{-1} day). Two skin biopsies were taken during the past year. The first biopsy showed neutrophilic dermatitis, folliculitis and furunculosis. The second biopsy, taken 8 months later, showed chronic pyogranulomatous dermatitis and follicular rupture. Antibiotics have been given for 26 weeks of the past year.

Questions

1. Describe the abnormalities and pertinent normal features in Figures 7.1–7.5.
2. What differential diagnoses should be considered for this presentation?
3. What tests could you perform to make the diagnosis?

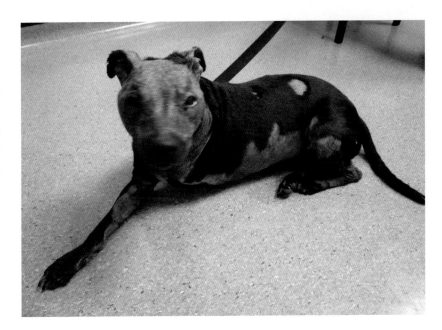

Figure 7.1

Small Animal Dermatology: What's Your Diagnosis? First Edition. Jane Coatesworth.
© 2019 John Wiley & Sons, Inc. Published 2019 by John Wiley & Sons, Inc.

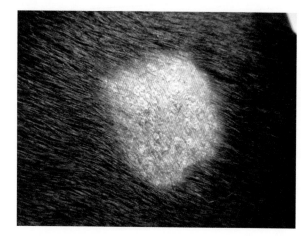

Figure 7.2

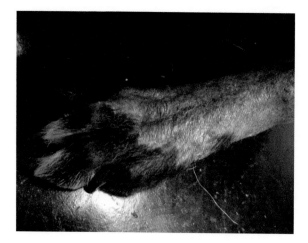

Figure 7.3

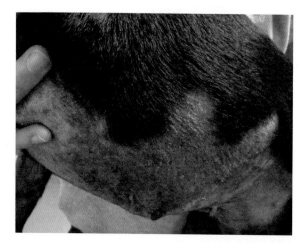

Figure 7.4

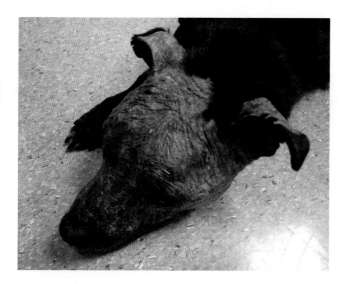

Figure 7.5

Answers

1. **What the figures show**

   Figure 7.1 shows a bright and alert dog. She has large, well-demarcated, areas of alopecia affecting the trunk, head and limbs. Hair loss affects approximately 50% of the surface area of the skin.

   Figure 7.2 shows the left hip area. There is a circular patch of alopecia with mildly erythematous skin, overlaid by a moderate amount of silvery grey scale. The adjacent hair coat has a normal appearance.

   Figure 7.3 shows the distal aspect of the left hind limb. All three limbs have large patches of alopecia. The affected skin has areas of erythema and hyperpigmentation. There is scale exfoliated onto the table top.

   Figure 7.4 shows the lateral body wall. There is a large area of inflamed erythematous skin, with overlying scale, caudal to the remaining hair coat. Note the sharply contrasting margins, abutting normal grey skin, both caudally and adjacent to the owner's ungloved hand. The affected skin is particularly erythematous at the margins.

   Figure 7.5 shows the head from above. The skin is totally alopecic, including the eyelashes, whiskers and the base of both pinnae. There is a healing area of excoriation over the left zygomatic arch. The skin is hyperpigmented, thickened and has areas of overlying silvery scale.

2. **Differential diagnoses**

   Given the appearance of the skin lesions the following conditions should be considered:

   - Demodicosis. Adult-onset generalised demodicosis can be seen in association with immunosuppression. This dog has a recent history of major surgery and neoplasia, she has also received daily glucocorticoids for the past 6 months. No mites were seen on skin biopsies, but this is a relatively insensitive diagnostic tool for *Demodex*.
   - Dermatophytosis. One of the family members in the household has been treated by their family doctor for suspected ringworm over the past month.

3. **Appropriate diagnostic tests**

   Hair plucks. A high proportion of the plucked hairs have follicular casts. Follicular casts are commonly associated with both demodicosis and dermatophytosis. Hairs are pulled out from the edge of the alopecic areas. No *Demodex* mites are found on hair plucks. This does not exclude demodicosis, and skin scrapes are needed at this point. Plucks are usually performed before scraping as they often give a positive diagnosis, and are quicker and less invasive to perform.

Skin scrapes. *Demodex canis* mites live in the hair follicles, so scrapes need to be deep enough to sample this area. Multiple deep scrapes, with a blunted scalpel blade, remove some of the dermis and produce oozing from the skin capillaries. No *Demodex* mites are found in the scraped material.

Wood's lamp. No fluorescence of the hairs is seen. Only half of the isolates of *Microsporum canis* show the characteristic apple green fluorescence of infected hairs. This means that other strains of *M. canis*, a different *Microsporum*, or a *Trichophyton* species could be present and still give a negative Wood's lamp result.

Dermatophyte culture. Intact hairs are plucked from the margins of alopecic areas and sent to the laboratory for dermatophyte culture.

Initial treatment

The dog is washed all over in a miconazole/chlorhexidine shampoo twice a week while waiting for the results of dermatophyte culture.

Oral prednisolone is reduced from $1\,\mathrm{mg\,kg^{-1}}$ each day, to an alternating pattern of $1\,\mathrm{mg\,kg^{-1}}$ one day and $0.5\,\mathrm{mg\,kg^{-1}}$ the next. Members of the family are recommended to wash their hands after touching the dog.

Diagnosis

Microsporum canis is isolated on dermatophyte culture after 8 days.

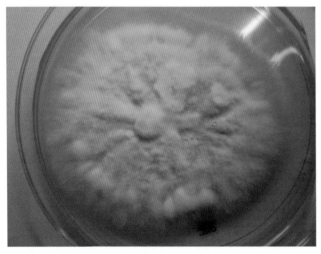

Figure 7.6 Shows a Petri dish containing Sabouraud's agar and a colony of the dermatophyte *M. canis*. Diagnostic features include a fluffy lemon-yellow and white appearance to the colony, with a lemon-yellow edge and radial grooves. The reverse (not shown) has a uniform yellow colour. Picking up some of the colony surface with adhesive tape shows macroconidia of an elongated lemon shape, and with more than six internal cells.

Treatment

Treatment will need to be continued until there are two negative fungal culture results 4 weeks apart.

Owner education and treatment effort is focussed on four main areas:

o Treatment of the dog. Itraconazole is given at 5 mg kg^{-1} once daily by mouth and with food.
o Reduce the shedding of spores from the dog in to the environment. Twice weekly bathing is continued with a miconazole/chlorhexidine shampoo.
o Reduce the number of spores in the environment. Use a vacuum cleaner regularly to pick up hair and skin scale. Remove all visible dirt with detergent, rinse and dry. Wipe down hard surfaces with dilute household bleach (1 : 30 dilution of a 0.5% solution) or with chlorhexidine (1 : 4 dilution of a 2% solution).
o Discuss the potential zoonotic risks with the owners.

After 3 weeks of treatment the erythema has resolved and the degree of scaling is much reduced.

After 5 weeks of treatment a sample taken for fungal culture grows *M. canis*. The fungal culture is positive after 6 days. The dose of prednisolone is tapered over a 5-week period and is then discontinued. The dog is no longer pruritic. There are a few patches of early hair regrowth on the abdomen and head. The frequency of oral itraconazole is reduced to alternate week dosing.

After 10 and 14 weeks of treatment. There is no growth on fungal culture from hair samples at either time point. All treatment is discontinued and the dog has no recurrence of active clinical signs. There is partial patchy hair regrowth at the previously alopecic areas. Persistent alopecia is particularly noticeable over the face, which was one of the first areas to be affected.

Prognosis

The prognosis is good if the dog has a sufficiently competent cell mediated immunity, and if enough cleaning has occurred to significantly reduce the re-infection challenge from spores in the environment. Dermatophyte cases normally develop a short-lived immunity to re-infection.

Discussion

Generalised dermatophytosis is uncommon in mature dogs and cats, and raises the suspicion of concurrent immune compromise as is likely in this case. The alopecia in this case started around the time of major surgery and the diagnosis of neoplasia. The dermatophyte infection was probably unable to self-cure due to the relatively high daily doses of prednisolone given over the past 6 months and the dogs' inability to mount an adequate inflammatory response. The ability to mount a competent cell mediated response is important for clearing a dermatophyte infection, and for providing short-term protection against re-infection. The clinical signs in a case of dermatophytosis are a balance between the virulence of the isolate and species of dermatophyte, and the degree and nature of the individual host response.

A diagnosis of dermatophytosis is based on positive fungal culture, positive Wood's lamp fluorescence, or fungal elements seen on skin biopsy or direct microscopy, in combination with suggestive clinical signs. Ideally direct microscopy, Wood's lamp examination or histopathology are positive in a case, as these three investigations demonstrate fungal elements within the hair shaft. Fungal culture only shows whether or not there are fungal spores on the hair coat, not whether the fungal spores are associated with a true infection. Diagnosis can be difficult as the clinical signs of dermatophytosis are highly variable, histopathology may not reveal the invading hyphae, as in this case, and fungal culture can give both false positive and false negative results. Despite the difficulties it is important to pursue a definitive diagnosis due to the zoonotic risk, the potential toxicity of the triazole treatment, and the significant cost and effort of the lengthy treatment period.

Dermatophytosis is generally treated until there are two negative fungal culture results, 4 weeks apart. The first sample for repeat fungal culture is generally taken 4–6 weeks into treatment. The chronic nature of this case, and the pyogranulomatous changes seen on histopathology, make it unsurprising that there is still a positive result on fungal culture after the first 5 weeks of treatment.

Itraconazole is highly bound to keratin, the structural protein that makes up skin, hair and claws. The high degree of binding makes itraconazole a good choice for the systemic treatment of dermatophytosis and allows it to be given as a pulse therapy, such as the 'one week on, one week off' treatment used here. There is enhanced absorption of itraconazole from the gastrointestinal tract when the capsule formulation is given with food. Interestingly, in people, the liquid formulation of itraconazole is better absorbed in the absence of food. A licensed liquid formulation of itraconazole is available in the UK for cats, and is also suitable for the treatment small dogs with informed consent from the owner. Itraconazole is converted into inactive metabolites by the liver. It may cause elevations in liver enzymes and is contraindicated with hepatic disease. The most common adverse effect of itraconazole is anorexia, but this is usually mild and the drug is generally well tolerated by dogs.

Microsporum canis, Trichophyton mentagrophytes and *Microsporum gypseum* are thought to be the most common dermatophyte species that cause disease in dogs. They infect the hair follicles and the hair shafts. Infected hair shafts are brittle and break into fragments, each containing high numbers of spores. The infectious arthrospores can survive for months or even years in the environment, hence the importance of topical treatment and environmental cleansing.

Clipping the hair coat can remove large amounts of infected hairs and infectious spores from the animal and prevent them from contaminating the environment. Clipped hair needs to be carefully collected and disposed of and the clippers disinfected after use. Microtrauma to the skin from clipping can allow more extensive dermatophyte lesions to develop. The use of a fixed length atraumatic stand-off, when clipping long haired dogs, can reduce the incidence of skin trauma. This dog, with its short and partial hair coat, was not clipped.

Both histopathology reports, from skin biopsies taken on two occasions, pointed towards folliculitis and subsequent furunculosis, follicular rupture and pyogranulomatous dermatitis. The three causes of folliculitis in the dog and cat – bacterial folliculitis, demodicosis and dermatophytosis – are often not identified on skin biopsy, separate and specific diagnostic tests are needed to rule them in or out of the differential list. It is unlikely that this dog ever had a bacterial skin infection. Receiving speculative oral antibiotics for 6 months is costly for the client, unhelpful for the dog and likely to contribute to the development of resistant bacteria.

Further reading

Cabanes, F.J., Abarca, M.L., and Bragulat, M.R. (1997). Dermatophytes isolated from domestic animals in Barcelona, Spain. *Mycopathologia* 137: 107–113.

Moriello, K., Coyner, K., Paterson, S., and Mignon, B. (2017). Diagnosis and treatment of dermatophytosis in dogs and cats. Clinical consensus guidelines of the World Association for Veterinary Dermatology. *Veterinary Dermatology* 28: 266–303.

History

A 2 ½ year-old male neutered Airedale Terrier is presented with a history of immune-mediated polyarthritis. He has received prednisolone, at $0.3\,\mathrm{mg\,kg^{-1}}$ once daily, for more than 1 year, and a higher dose for the 6 months prior to that. The owner first noticed a bilaterally symmetrical non-pruritic flank alopecia 2 months before treatment started for the immune-mediated disease. Two months after starting prednisolone the alopecic flank patches enlarged. There was slowly progressive thinning of the coat over the trunk, then the tail and then the pinnae. The dog has recently been biting at the right hind paw.

Questions

1. Describe the abnormalities and pertinent normal features in Figures 8.1–8.5.
2. What differential diagnoses should be considered for this presentation?
3. What tests could you perform to make the diagnosis?

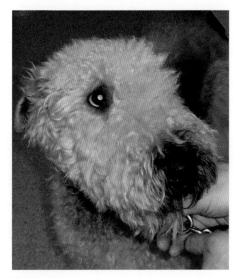

Figure 8.1

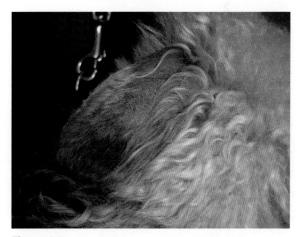

Figure 8.2

Small Animal Dermatology: What's Your Diagnosis? First Edition. Jane Coatesworth.
© 2019 John Wiley & Sons, Inc. Published 2019 by John Wiley & Sons, Inc.

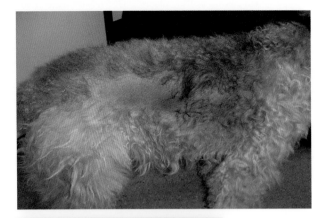

Figure 8.3

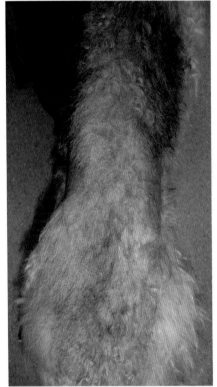

Figure 8.4

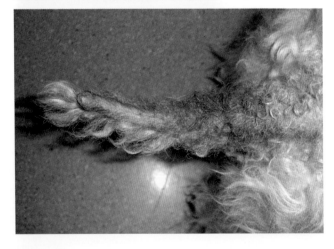

Figure 8.5

Answers

1. What the figures show

Figure 8.1 shows an abnormally pale coloured soft and fluffy hair coat over the head.

Figure 8.2 shows the left pinna. There is extensive alopecia at the base of the pinna. The right pinna is affected in a similar way.

Figure 8.3 shows the right side of the torso. There is an extensive alopecic patch on the right lateral thorax and flank. The alopecia is total at the caudal segment of the patch, and partial at the cranial part. The alopecic skin is developing hyperpigmentation.

Figure 8.4 shows the back and rump from above. There is hypotrichosis over the dorsal midline and pelvic area, and bilaterally symmetrical alopecia over the trunk. The remaining hair coat is generally soft, fluffy and pale in colour.

Figure 8.5 shows alopecia of the distal tail.

2. Differential diagnoses

Given the appearance of the skin lesions the following conditions should be considered:

- Canine flank alopecia. The Airedale Terrier, along with the Boxer and English Bulldog, is a predisposed breed. Non-pruritic bilaterally symmetrical alopecia, limited to the flanks, was the first clinical sign when the dog was 10 months of age. The dog is now 2½ years old and there has been no spontaneous hair regrowth in the intervening time.
- Hyperadrenocorticism – iatrogenic or spontaneous. The history of daily oral glucocorticoid treatment over a prolonged period, and the young age of onset of clinical signs, makes iatrogenic hyperadrenocorticism (HAC) more likely than spontaneous disease.
- Hypothyroidism can be a cause of non-pruritic bilaterally symmetrical alopecia, but is more common in older dogs with additional clinical signs. The thin and inelastic skin on the ventral abdomen would not be typical of hypothyroidism.
- Sex hormone alopecia.
- Demodicosis.
- Dermatophytosis is a potential cause of non-pruritic alopecia, but the changes in coat colour and texture, and the symmetrical pattern of alopecia would be unusual.

3. Appropriate diagnostic tests

Physical examination shows thin and inelastic skin of the ventral abdomen. Digit 2 of the right hind is swollen, with crusting around the nail fold and hyperpigmentation.

Orthopaedic examination shows no palpable joint effusions, but some discomfort on hip extension.

Hair plucks from the affected digit and from around the eyes show high numbers of *Demodex* mites in all life stages. The overpopulation of *Demodex* mites in this case is likely to be a consequence of the long term steroid usage. Although the digit was most severely affected, *Demodex* mites were easily found elsewhere on the body.

Cytology from the affected digit shows neutrophils with intra and extracytoplasmic cocci, suggestive of bacterial pyoderma.

Diagnosis

Canine flank alopecia, which is common in this breed, followed by iatrogenic hyperadrenocorticism secondary to the daily administration of prednisolone, and subsequent generalised demodicosis. It is possible that the initial non-pruritic alopecia was caused by juvenile onset demodicosis, but the bilaterally symmetrical flank distribution would be unusual for demodicosis.

Treatment

The oral prednisolone is reduced to a staggered alternate day therapy, that is, giving 0.3 mg kg^{-1} one day and 0.15 mg kg^{-1} the next day, for 2 weeks. Amitraz is recommended for weekly application to the whole body. The right hind paw is washed in a chlorhexidine based shampoo every other day.

Prognosis

The prognosis for iatrogenic hyperadrenocorticism is good if no further glucocorticoids are given, or if they are given in a sustainable fashion (usually up to 0.5 mg kg^{-1} every other day). Changes in the skin and hair coat are entirely reversible once glucocorticoids are discontinued.

The immune-mediated polyarthritis may recur and, if it does, the prognosis depends on what type and dosage of drugs may be needed to keep it in remission. If the polyarthritis does not recur the prognosis is good. It is likely, in this case, that the prednisolone was a significant factor for the demodicosis. Without prednisolone the dog's immune system is likely to be able to maintain the population of *Demodex* mites at a subclinical level. Some cases of juvenile onset generalised demodicosis require ongoing intermittent treatment to maintain the *Demodex* population at a low level.

The prognosis for canine flank alopecia is good, as it is a localised cosmetic condition. The pattern of hair loss and regrowth is very variable.

Final outcome

The *Demodex* numbers fell to zero on subsequent hair plucks and then on deep skin scrapes over a period of 7 weeks. The oral prednisolone was slowly reduced, and discontinued after an 8-week taper, that is, 0.3 mg kg^{-1} every other day for 2 weeks, then 0.15 mg kg^{-1} every other day for 2 weeks, then 0.08 mg kg^{-1} every other day for 2 weeks, then stop.

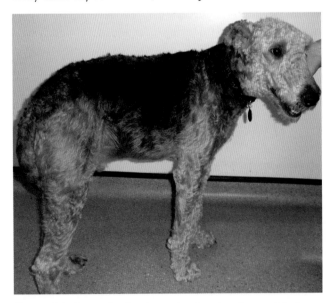

Figure 8.6 Shows the dog 4 months after stopping prednisolone. There is good hair regrowth at all of the previously alopecic areas. The new hair coat has the lustre, colour and crimped texture typical of an Airedale Terrier, and is significantly different in texture and appearance to the previous hair coat. The flank areas, which have been persistently alopecic since 10 months of age, have also regrown a full hair coat. It will be interesting to see if this is subsequently shed, consistent with the typical cyclic pattern of canine flank alopecia.

Discussion

Amitraz was used in this case to successfully reduce *Demodex* mite numbers. An isoxazoline drug is a more convenient choice, now that these drugs are available and licensed for use in demodicosis.

The duration of the demodicosis is unknown in this case, and demodicosis is a non-pruritic condition in the dog. The recently observed biting at the right hind paw, along with the clinical signs of inflammation, suggest a recent secondary bacterial folliculitis at this site. This is confirmed by the intracytoplasmic cocci seen on cytology from the swollen digit. Topical therapy with regular chlorhexidine washes, in combination with treatment for *Demodex*, allowed the bacterial folliculitis to resolve. Systemic antibiotics are not indicated in this instance.

The dose of prednisolone ($0.3\,\mathrm{mg\,kg^{-1}}$) was in the low anti-inflammatory range, but the daily administration over a prolonged period led to adverse effects. The hair coat was showing signs of telogen arrest; for example, the inability to regrow hair at alopecic areas, faded hair colour, a dull lustreless coat and a soft fluffy hair texture. Daily corticosteroids, even at low doses, can suppress the hypothalamic pituitary axis and lead to iatrogenic HAC. The normal pulsatile production of corticosteroids from the adrenal glands is lost, and the dog becomes dependent on the exogenous source. Despite the low starting dose, the oral steroids were tapered slowly in this case. A slow taper reduces the risk of an Addisonian crisis, and allows time for endogenous corticosteroid production to resume.

Further reading

Miller, M. and Dunstan, R. (1993). Seasonal flank alopecia in Boxers and Airedale Terriers. *Journal of the American Veterinary Medical Association* 203: 1567–1572.

Pigmentation

Normal pigmentation

The colour of the skin and hair coat is dependent on the amount, distribution and the type of melanin present. The normal pattern of distribution of melanin within the skin or hair shaft is genetically determined. The pigment eumelanin gives rise to black and brown coloration, while phaeomelanin gives rise to red and yellow. An absence of pigment results in pink skin and/or a white hair coat. Melanin is synthesised inside melanocytes, from the amino acid tyrosine.

$$\text{Tyrosine} \xrightarrow{\text{Tyrosinase}} \text{Dopa} \rightarrow \text{Melanins}$$

Melanocytes are found in the hair bulbs and in the basal layer of the epidermis. Melanin is produced and packaged inside melanosomes and then transported down the elongated 'arms' of the melanocytes. The tips of the dendritic 'arms' of the melanocytes are in contact with keratinocytes. Melanosomes are transferred across from the melanocytes to the keratinocytes and confer specific colour to the skin or hair.

Melanin is able to absorb and dissipate most of the energy of ultraviolet radiation and largely protects pigmented skin from radiation damage. Ultraviolet radiation is potentially damaging to the skin and DNA is particularly vulnerable to radiation damage. Melanin pigment is orientated in a protective cap over the nucleus within each nucleated keratinocyte. The degree of exposure to ultraviolet radiation depends on the lifestyle and skin type of the individual, the nature of the hair coat, the time of year, the latitude and the local weather conditions. Areas with a sparse hair coat and inadequate pigmentation are especially vulnerable to radiation damage and the potential consequences such as squamous cell carcinoma.

Abnormal pigmentation of the skin and coat can manifest as an increase or decrease in pigmentation or as a change in colour.

Increased pigmentation

This can be *genetic*, for example, lentigo on the lips and nose of a ginger or tortoiseshell cat, or on the trunk of a Pug. Lentigines are hyperpigmented macules. The skin is flat and there is no associated inflammation. *Post-inflammatory*, for example, after bacterial or *Malassezia* infection, or in allergic skin disease. Inflammation in the epidermis causes melanocytes to increase their production of melanin and to transfer melanin to the surrounding keratinocytes. Post-inflammatory hyperpigmentation, in contrast to hypopigmentation, tends to be a consequence of less severe inflammation and to be a reversible change.

Small Animal Dermatology: What's Your Diagnosis? First Edition. Jane Coatesworth.
© 2019 John Wiley & Sons, Inc. Published 2019 by John Wiley & Sons, Inc.

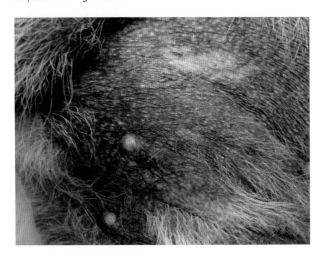

Figure B.1 Shows the ventral abdomen of a young Golden Retriever with atopic dermatitis. There is marked hyperpigmentation and lichenification of the glabrous skin.

Ultraviolet induced, for example, in areas of skin without an adequate protective hair coat.

Pigmented tumours, for example, most melanomas, basal cell tumours. These are usually raised above the surrounding normal skin as a physical mass. Fine needle aspirate and biopsy are needed to distinguish from benign masses such as melanocytic naevi.

Associated with *hormonal diseases*, for example, hyperadrenocorticism or hypothyroidism. Hyperpigmented macules can occur in association with endocrinopathies and testicular tumours.

Decreased pigmentation
Genetic

Albinism is an autosomal recessive trait, caused by a mutation in the tyrosinase gene. Albinos have melanocytes but no functional tyrosinase and are unable to produce melanin. In dogs and cats the irides appear blue, the skin pink and the hair coat white.

Colour points

Siamese cats, with darker coloured extremities, also have a mutation of the tyrosinase gene. The mutation makes expression of the gene dependent on the temperature of the skin. Warm areas of the body have less gene expression and are a paler shade, while the 'points' have normal expression of tyrosinase and are dark coloured.

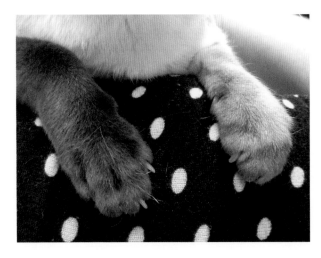

Figure B.2 Shows the front paws of a Siamese cat. The left fore paw has a chronic inflammatory skin disease and a persistently elevated temperature, leading to a paler hair coat colour. The right fore paw shows the normal darker colour. The left fore paw reverted to the normal dark colour when the inflammation finally resolved.

Congenital coat-colour-related neurosensory deafness

Neural crest cells (melanocyte precursors) normally migrate to the proto-ear at an early stage of development. Functional melanocytes, located in the inner ear, are important for hearing. Failure of melanocyte migration, or of maturation, can result in complete deafness in one or both ears. Deaf puppies or kittens often have blue eyes and a merle or largely white hair coat on the head. Interestingly, the white ear is not necessarily the deaf one. Brain auditory evoked response (BAER) testing is helpful to accurately diagnose deafness. The condition is seen in the dog, cat, horse, llama and alpaca. A variety of dog breeds are affected, such as the Dalmatian, Border Collie, English Bull Terrier and Australian Shepherd.

Immune mediated

Melanocytes may be directly targeted by auto-antibodies leading to damage or death of the pigment producing cells. This occurs in conditions such as vitiligo and uveodermatologic syndrome. The strong breed associations for these diseases suggest a genetic influence, but their spontaneous appearance in a range of atypical breeds suggests either a random mutation or that other factors are influential.

Acquired

Post-inflammatory loss of pigment from the skin and hair coat tends to follow severe inflammation. There may be permanent depigmentation, due to destruction of melanocytes during the inflammatory process.

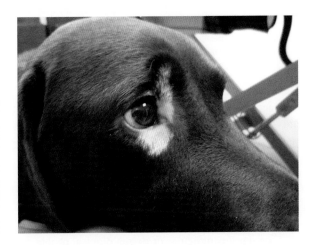

Figure B.3 Shows a young chocolate Labrador Retriever with a large patch of leucotrichia ventral and rostral to the right eye. The affected area of coat was previously alopecic and severely inflamed. The changes followed an adverse reaction to a topical ocular medication.

Pigmentary incontinence

Inflammation of the interface between the dermis and epidermis can allow pigment to cross from the epidermis into the dermis, where it is usually engulfed by macrophages. This type of pigment loss from the epidermis can be a feature of pemphigus foliaceus, epitheliotropic lymphoma and discoid lupus erythematosus. When pigment is lost from the epidermis in this way the skin often has a slate blue/grey appearance where it was previously black.

Colour change

An area of *red skin* can be caused by inflammation or by haemorrhage into the skin. With inflammation there is increased blood flow to the area and the blood is within the blood vessels. When haemorrhage occurs into the skin, the blood escapes from the blood vessels into the surrounding tissue. The resulting red area of skin can look similar in both cases and diascopy, using a glass slide pressed firmly onto the skin surface, helps to tell them apart. The colour of the skin under the slide is compared to the colour of the surrounding lesional skin. If the pressed area blanches, the red blood is being pushed out of the area. To be able to move quickly, away from the pressure, the blood must be inside blood vessels and the lesion is therefore inflammatory. If the pressed area stays red, the blood cannot easily escape from the pressure and must be outside of the blood vessels. The lesion is therefore not just inflammatory and may be associated with leaky blood vessels (vasculitis), or with reduced blood clotting ability.

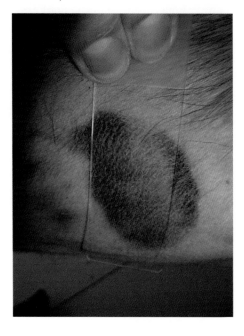

Figure B.4 Shows a glass slide firmly pressed onto a discoloured area of skin. The skin beneath the slide is not blanched, suggesting that a proportion of the red blood cells are outside of blood vessels. This dog has a vasculopathy.

The skin can have a diffuse *yellow colour* (jaundice) when an animal has significantly elevated blood levels of bilirubin. Bilirubin is a breakdown product of haemoglobin and is largely metabolised by the liver. Jaundice is most readily recognised on the sclerae and on the concave pinnae and gums, provided that the skin is not heavily pigmented. Common underlying causes of jaundice are haemolysis, hepatopathy and bile duct obstruction.

Reddish brown staining of light coloured hair coat can be a result of tear staining; for example, at the medial canthus of the eye when there is tear overflow onto the face. Staining is also seen associated with excessive licking; for example, stained front feet in a dog with atopic dermatitis. The characteristic reddish brown colour is associated with porphyrins, which can be found in canine saliva, tears and urine. While the staining is only a cosmetic problem it can be a marker for significant ocular or dermatological problems, and possible underlying causes should always be investigated.

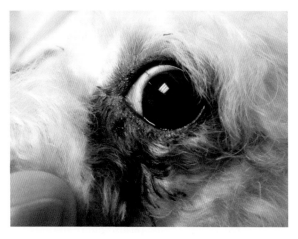

Figure B.5 Shows the left eye of a 5 year-old female neutered Bichon Frise. The dog has red/brown staining at the medial canthus associated with persistent excess tearing.

History

A 2 year-old male neutered English springer spaniel presents with a 6-month history of dryness, and some cracking, of the nasal planum. The skin changes are first noticed 6 months ago and have steadily progressed. The owner reports that the dog is unaffected by the condition, and shows no signs of illness, pruritus or discomfort. The dog is fully vaccinated and dewormed, and has not travelled outside of the United Kingdom. There has been no previous treatment.

Questions

1. Describe the abnormalities and pertinent normal features in Figure 9.1.
2. What differential diagnoses should be considered for this presentation?
3. What tests could you perform to make the diagnosis?

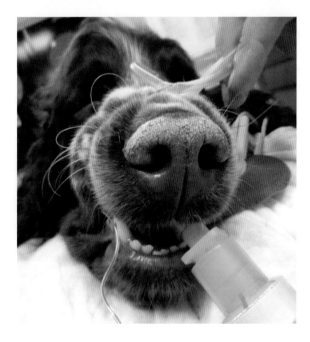

Figure 9.1

Answers

1. **What the figures show**

Figure 9.1 shows the nasal planum with the dog under anaesthetic at the time of skin biopsy. The entire nasal planum is swollen and the nasal philtrum is exaggerated ventrally. There is loss of the normal cobblestone surface architecture. There is adherent yellow crust over the dorsal half of the nasal planum, and a number of vertical fissures radiating dorsally from the nostrils. The entire nasal planum is depigmented to a pink colour. There is a sharp demarcation between the affected nasal planum and the adjacent normal skin, and hair coat, of the rostral muzzle. The changes to the nasal planum are bilaterally symmetrical.

Small Animal Dermatology: What's Your Diagnosis? First Edition. Jane Coatesworth.
© 2019 John Wiley & Sons, Inc. Published 2019 by John Wiley & Sons, Inc.

2. Differential diagnoses

Given the appearance of the skin lesions the following conditions should be considered:

- Discoid lupus erythematosus (DLE). This is the most common inflammatory disease of the nasal planum in the dog. Individual cases vary in severity, from mild and cosmetic to extensive and severe.
- Localised pemphigus foliaceus, or pemphigus erythematosus. These two conditions can have a similar clinical appearance to DLE, especially when erosion and ulceration are present. Histopathology is usually helpful in telling them apart.
- Vitiligo. This is unlikely as the dog has no pigment loss affecting the hair coat and vitiligo does not show clinical signs of inflammation.
- Idiopathic nasal depigmentation. This is usually a cyclic and seasonal condition. There is partial to complete nasal depigmentation, occurring mainly in the winter. In contrast to this case there is no associated inflammation, and the normal nasal architecture is unaffected. Labrador Retrievers, Poodles and Golden Retrievers are predisposed, but other breeds can be affected.
- Uveodermatologic syndrome. This is unlikely as the eyes are unaffected, the dog has no pigment loss affecting the hair coat and the English springer spaniel is not a predisposed breed.
- Mucocutaneous pyoderma (MCP). This condition resolves with antibiotics and is usually seen around the lips. The mucocutaneous junctions of the nasal planum can be affected. Unlike DLE, the lesions are not usually symmetrical.
- Systemic lupus erythematosus (SLE). This could present with identical clinical and histopathological changes of the nasal planum, to those seen in DLE, but the dog has no systemic signs of disease (e.g. anaemia, thrombocytopenia and polyarthritis).
- Leishmaniosis. This dog has no travel history, but several cases of leishmaniosis have been reported in the UK where the affected dog has not been out of the country. The UK does not currently have the sand fly (*Phlebotomus*), which is the usual vector for *Leishmania spp*. Leishmaniosis is a particularly important differential when there are ulcerated and/or erosive lesions on the nasal planum. In the absence of visible *Leishmania* parasites, the histopathological findings in leishmaniosis, MCP and DLE can all have a similar appearance.

3. Appropriate diagnostic tests

Haematology and serum biochemistry are unremarkable. These tests are helpful to screen for changes associated with SLE, for example thrombocytopenia, anaemia and neutropenia. Haematology and serum biochemistry provide useful baseline values for comparison with future blood samples, especially if they are taken before any medication is given.

Skin biopsies. The nasal planum can be a challenging place to biopsy. There is a tendency for a lot of bleeding. The closure of biopsy sites needs firm but gentle suture pressure to give appropriate apposition and to avoid the sutures cutting free. The area is very sensitive and self-trauma of the healing biopsy sites can lead to wound breakdown. Areas with slate blue/grey coloration, with no ulceration or erosion, are ideal biopsy sites.

It is helpful to take skin biopsies after 2–3 weeks of systemic antibiotics, if MCP is considered to be a significant differential diagnosis. The clinical signs of MCP will clear completely with an appropriate course of antibiotics. In contrast, the clinical signs of DLE are unaffected by antibiotics or are only partially improved by the resolution of a secondary bacterial pyoderma. It is important to use an antibiotic such as cephalexin for this treatment trial, rather than one with immune modulating effects such as a tetracycline.

Histopathology shows infiltration of the superficial dermis with large numbers of plasma cells, lymphocytes and neutrophils and occasional macrophages. The dermal-epidermal junction is indistinct in places, with vacuolar degeneration of basal cells. Apoptotic (shrunken and eosinophilic) epithelial cells are present in the stratum spinosum and stratum basale. There is a moderate amount of compact parakeratotic hyperkeratosis.

Diagnosis
The clinical signs and histopathology are consistent with DLE.

Treatment
This case shows the localised form of DLE so topical treatment, with tacrolimus 0.1% ointment, is recommended. Owners need to wear gloves when applying tacrolimus. Unfortunately, the dog is uncooperative and it is not possible for the owner to apply any topical treatment. Topical tacrolimus gives an unpleasant burning or tingling skin sensation in some people. In this case the lack of patient cooperation was not due to an adverse effect of the tacrolimus, as the drug never touched the nose!

The dog is given the immunomodulatory combination of oral oxytetracycline (500 mg every 8 hours) and niacinamide (500 mg every 8 hours). There is a good reduction in swelling and adherent crust after 1 month of treatment. The pigmentation of the nasal planum, and the 'cobblestone' surface contour, return gradually over a 6-month period. The owner comments that the dog is brighter and is working better, suggesting retrospectively that the active disease was having some impact on wellbeing.

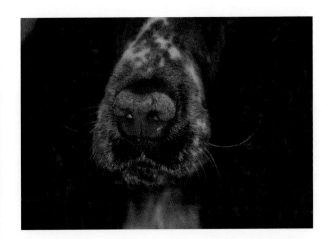

Figure 9.2 Shows the nose after 12 days of oral medication. The skin underlying the crusted areas, and down the philtrum, has a pale pink to grey appearance and some reduction in swelling. The rest of the nasal planum skin is erythematous and swollen to the same degree as before.

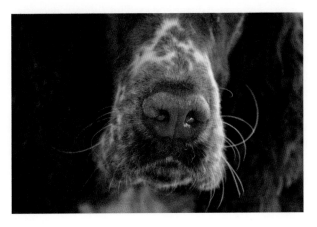

Figure 9.3 Shows the nose after 25 days of oral medication. There is a significant reduction in swelling of the nasal planum, allowing the nasal philtrum to have a more normal appearance. There is a reduced amount of yellow crust over the dorsal aspect of the nasal planum. The surface contour of the skin is smooth, with persistent loss of the normal cobblestone appearance. The vertical fissures, which are only present in the dorsal section of the nasal planum, are less pronounced.

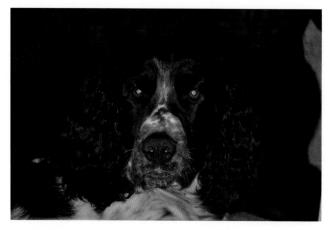

Figure 9.4 Shows the dog after five months of receiving medication. There is a significant amount of re-pigmentation and the normal cobblestone pattern of the skin surface has largely returned. The nose is not swollen and the dog appears to be completely comfortable. This photograph was taken in the winter, so reduced ultraviolet exposure may also be contributing to the improvement in clinical signs.

Prognosis

The prognosis is good, with ongoing treatment and the avoidance of excessive ultraviolet light.

Discussion

DLE is part of the cutaneous lupus erythematosus (CLE) family of skin diseases. DLE is the most commonly occurring disease out of the CLE group. The condition is aggravated by ultraviolet light and there is a tendency for flares of disease activity to occur during the summer months. Topical sunscreen is a useful option in some patients, but would not have been possible in this case. Clinical signs started in February. The dog was presented in July, when clinical signs were at their most severe and the condition improved in September. This pattern may reflect ultraviolet light levels, a response to treatment or an innate fluctuation in disease severity.

The CLE diseases have characteristic microscopic features on histopathology. These include inflammation of the deep epidermis and the superficial dermis (interface dermatitis). The infiltration of lymphocytes and plasma cells to these areas may obscure the dermal-epidermal junction. Cytotoxic T-lymphocytes cause damage, especially to the basal layer of the epidermis. Increased numbers of keratinocytes in the basal layer die, either by programmed cell death (apoptosis) or by membrane damage and swelling (oncotic necrosis). The melanocytes, sitting on the basement membrane, can be damaged and pigment can pass through into the dermis where it is engulfed by macrophages. These changes, called pigmentary incontinence, are seen clinically as a skin colour change to slate blue/grey.

The lesions, in this case, are restricted to the nasal planum. This is the initial lesion location in most cases of localised DLE, often starting at the junction of the haired skin and the dorsal nasal planum. Lesions may subsequently involve the dorso-rostral muzzle, the lips, around the eyes and the pinnae. Less commonly the vulva, footpads and perineum are affected. A rare generalised form of DLE presents with lesions on the head, neck, trunk and proximal limbs. DLE is reported in a wide range of breeds. The localised form is mostly seen in breeds with a longer muzzle conformation, such as the German Shepherd dog and Collie.

The clinical signs of DLE are typically loss of pigmentation, loss of normal architecture, swelling, erosion and ulceration of the nasal planum. Significant ulceration of the nasal planum can be associated with recurrent haemorrhage. This case shows loss of pigmentation, loss of normal architecture and swelling, there is no ulceration or erosion. Mucocutaneous areas, such as the lips, eyelids and vulva, can show similar clinical signs. When haired skin is affected, the lesions are approximately circular macules and plaques, with adherent scaling and hyper or hypopigmentation. The lesions can be erythematous and eroded and chronic lesions can have central scarring alopecia. Dogs with DLE are systemically well, but may have absent to mild pruritus and discomfort associated with the skin lesions.

This dog is treated with the immunomodulatory combination of oxytetracycline and niacinamide. The tetracyclines, including oxytetracycline, have both antibacterial and immunomodulatory properties. The long-term use of antibiotics can contribute to the selection of resistant bacteria, so finding alternative treatments is desirable. Other reported treatment options for localised DLE include systemic and/or topical corticosteroids, oral vitamin E and essential fatty acid supplementation. Topical corticosteroids are not an option in this dog due to poor patient cooperation. Systemic corticosteroids are not considered to be an appropriate choice in this case. The risk of potential adverse effects, including behavioural changes and exacerbation of aggression, are felt to outweigh the benefits to this localised condition.

Cases of generalised DLE have been successfully treated with systemic tetracycline and niacinamide, ciclosporin or corticosteroids. Hydroxychloroquine, an antimalarial drug, has been used at 5 mg kg^{-1} orally once daily to treat generalised DLE, but did not give sustained control of the clinical signs.

Further reading

Banovic, F., Linder, K.E., Uri, M. et al. (2016). Clinical and microscopic features of generalized discoid lupus erythematosus in dogs (10 cases). *Veterinary Dermatology* 27: 488–499.

Banovic, F., Olivry, T., and Linder, K.E. (2014). Ciclosporin therapy for canine generalized discoid lupus erythematosus refractory to doxycycline and niacinamide. *Veterinary Dermatology* 25: 483–486.

Griffies, J.D., Mendelsohn, C.L., Rosenkrantz, W.S. et al. (2004). Topical 0.1% tacrolimus for the treatment of discoid lupus erythematosus and pemphigus erythematosus. *Journal of the American Animal Hospital Association* 40: 29–41.

Oberkirchner, U., Linder, K.E., and Olivry, T. (2012). Successful treatment of a novel generalized variant of canine discoid lupus erythematosus with oral hydroxychloroquine. *Veterinary Dermatology* 23: 65–70.

History

A 10 year-old male neutered Shih Tzu presents with a 1-year history of itchy skin without apparent skin lesions. The other, unrelated, dog in the household is not pruritic. Both dogs are up to date with deworming and routine vaccinations and have monthly fipronil spot-on for flea control. The full litter brother, of the affected dog, is known by the owners and has no skin problems. Skin lesions are first noticed 2 months ago on the ventral neck, chest and axillae. The skin is red and scaly, and the dog scratches and rubs these areas to the point of bleeding. Cytology is supportive of a bacterial superficial pyoderma. The degree of pruritus reduces significantly after 4 weeks of oral cephalexin, at 21 mg kg^{-1} every 12 hours. The dog is diagnosed with demodicosis and has eight 0.05% w/v amitraz rinses at 1-week intervals. Two days after each of the first five amitraz rinses the dog is washed in a chlorhexidine/miconazole shampoo, as the owner feels the amitraz leads to increased pruritus. The dog is lethargic for 48 hours after each amitraz rinse. Two weeks ago the level of pruritus increases again, and is unresponsive to a 2-week course of oral cephalexin. The dog licks all four paws, scratches his neck and ears and shakes his head. His itch score is assessed by the owners as 6/10, when a normal dog would be 1/10.

Questions

1. Describe the abnormalities and pertinent normal features in Figures 10.1–10.3.
2. What differential diagnoses should be considered for this presentation?
3. What tests could you perform to make the diagnosis?

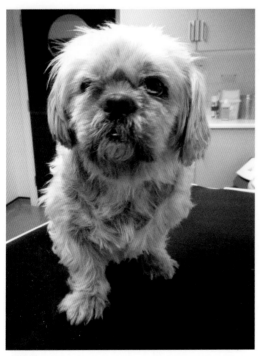

Figure 10.1

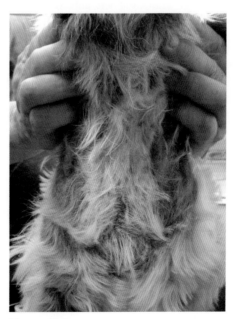

Figure 10.2

Small Animal Dermatology: What's Your Diagnosis? First Edition. Jane Coatesworth.
© 2019 John Wiley & Sons, Inc. Published 2019 by John Wiley & Sons, Inc.

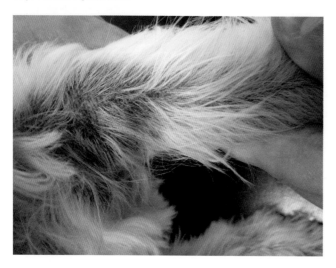

Figure 10.3

Answers

1. What the figures show

Figure 10.1 shows the subdued dog. There is hypotrichosis of the face and chest and hyperpigmentation of the underlying skin. The front nails are long and there is abnormal foot placement.

Figure 10.2 shows the ventral neck and chest, with the head elevated and the neck folds stretched laterally. There is a sparse hair coat. The non-pigmented skin is erythematous and the pigmented skin is hyperpigmented. There is a thick yellow material overlying the skin and matting the hair coat, at the rostral part of the ventral neck.

Figure 10.3 shows the left antecubital fossa. The hair coat is thin. The older long hairs are pale coloured, while the new shorter hairs are a pale brown colour. There is lichenification and hyperpigmentation of the skin.

2. Differential diagnoses

Given the appearance of the skin lesions the following conditions should be considered:

- Adult onset generalised demodicosis. This condition usually has an underlying immunosuppressive cause, such as endocrinopathy or neoplasia.
- *Malassezia* dermatitis. The commensal *Malassezia* yeasts on the skin commonly multiply and cause an overgrowth when the skin is inflamed.
- Bacterial superficial pyoderma. This is common secondary to demodicosis and the pruritus previously resolved after a 4-week course of antibiotics. However, no bacteria were found on cytology, and the dog had just had a 2-week course of antibiotics with no impact on the current level of pruritus.

3. Appropriate diagnostic tests

Physical examination shows marked enlargement of the prescapular and popliteal lymph nodes. The dog is inactive and has a depressed demeanour. The skin is generally greasy, especially in the axillae, groin and ventral neck, and there is associated malodour.

Cytology. Acetate tape strips from the skin show very high numbers of *Malassezia*, and no bacteria or inflammatory cells. Cytology on cotton bud swabs, from both ears, shows similar findings.

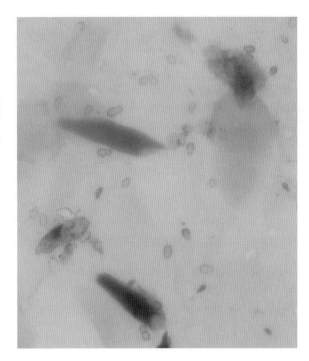

Figure 10.4 Was taken down the microscope and shows detail from an acetate tape strip preparation, which has been stained with methylene blue. The characteristic purple-staining 'snowman' shaped *Malassezia* are seen alongside large angular corneocytes. *Malassezia* are unipolar budding yeasts and the variable shapes represent the different stages of the budding process.

Hair plucks from the legs and face show numerous *Demodex canis* mites, in all life stages. Hair plucks are a less sensitive test for *Demodex* than skin scraping, but they are simpler, quicker, safer and less painful for the patient. If the hair plucks are negative then deep skin scrapes are needed to diagnose, or rule out, demodicosis. Skin biopsies can be necessary in the SharPei to diagnose demodicosis as excess mucin interferes with skin scraping.

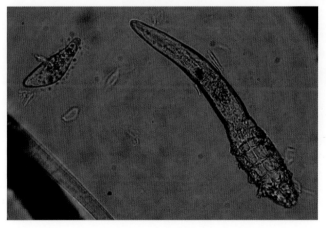

Figure 10.5 Was taken down the microscope, and shows detail from a hair pluck mounted in liquid paraffin. There is an eight-legged adult *Demodex canis* mite to the right of the image, and a lemon shaped *Demodex* egg on the left. A hair shaft gives a sense of relative scale, across the bottom left of the image.

Diagnosis
Adult onset generalised demodicosis, with *Malassezia* dermatitis and bilateral *Malassezia* otitis.
The underlying cause needs to be investigated.

Treatment and further investigations

There are still high numbers of *Demodex* mites on hair plucks, despite 8 weeks of treatment with amitraz. The efficacy of the drug is likely to have been diluted by the use of shampoo 2 days after application. Also, the skin is greasy and this may be a barrier to effective skin contact, and penetration down the hair follicles, by the amitraz. The chlorhexidine/miconazole shampoo used on the dog is likely to have helped to resolve the bacterial pyoderma, but does not have a degreasing action. The plan is to use an oral product to reduce the *Demodex* population, allowing for regular topical treatment of the skin greasiness and the high *Malassezia* population.

Oral fluralaner, at 42 mg kg^{-1}, is given now and in 3 months' time. This drug is not currently licensed for the treatment of demodicosis but it has shown good efficacy against raised populations of *Demodex* mites and is generally well tolerated.

The hair coat is clipped short to facilitate twice weekly bathing, once in a degreasing shampoo and once in a 3% chlorhexidine shampoo.

Treatment of the ears is delayed until they have been flushed and assessed.

Further diagnostic tests are performed 1 week later.

Radiographs of the right and left lateral thorax, and right lateral abdomen show no significant findings.

An ultrasound scan of the abdomen is unremarkable other than showing plump adrenal glands. This may reflect mild adrenal hyperplasia or pituitary dependent hyperadrenocorticism.

The radiographs and ultrasound scan are performed under general anaesthesia. While the dog is anaesthetised a large amount of dark brown debris is flushed from both ears, revealing intact and translucent tympanic membranes. The epithelial walls of the vertical and horizontal canals are mildly inflamed.

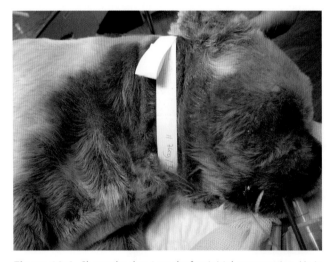

Figure 10.6 Shows the dog 1 week after initial presentation. He is under general anaesthetic and in left lateral recumbency. The hair coat has been clipped short to facilitate bathing. There is marked hyperpigmentation of the head and chest regions, with a sharp demarcation to normal skin on the left of the image. The dog has marked erythema of the concave aspect of the pinnae (visible on the right pinna).

A urine cortisol to creatinine ratio is 16×10^{-6}. The owner collected three consecutive morning urine samples at home. The samples were pooled and submitted for analysis. Results below 34×10^{-6} are considered to be within the normal range. This test has a low specificity and high sensitivity, so a result within the normal range can be used to rule out hyperadrenocorticism. A result above the normal range is not diagnostic for hyperadrenocorticism and further tests are needed to make a diagnosis.

The results of haematology and serum biochemistry are all unremarkable.

Final diagnosis and outcome

Adult onset generalised demodicosis, underlying cause unknown.

After 5 weeks of treatment the dog is much brighter, more playful and active. Hair plucks from the feet and ventral neck show one adult *Demodex* mite. Acetate tape strip cytology from the axillae and ventral neck, and cotton bud cytology from the ears, shows low numbers of *Malassezia*, no bacteria and no inflammatory cells. The skin and hair coat are not greasy and the dog is not malodorous. The itch score, assessed by the owners, is reduced to 1/10 and is similar to that of their other dog. The frequency of bathing is reduced to weekly, using the 3% chlorhexidine shampoo. The degreasing shampoo is discontinued.

A blood sample is taken for total T4 and thyroid stimulating hormone (TSH) assay and the results are unremarkable. This test is delayed until the dog appears to be well, as the results are commonly affected by non-thyroid illness.

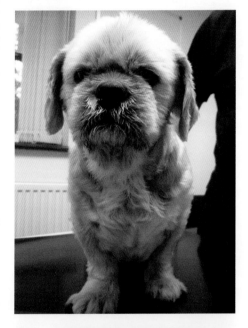

Figure 10.7 Shows the dog after 5 weeks of treatment. The dog has a brighter demeanour. The new hair coat is growing well and has a normal brown and white colour.

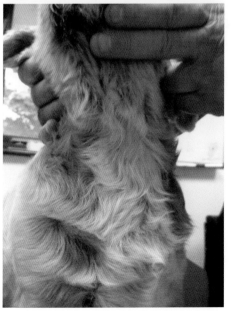

Figure 10.8 Shows the ventral neck and chest after 5 weeks of treatment. The non-pigmented skin of the ventral neck is now a normal pale pink colour. There is reduced hyperpigmentation of the pigmented areas. The skin and hair coat feel clean, dry, soft and smooth.

Prognosis

There is a good prognosis for a short-term reduction in the cutaneous *Demodex* and *Malassezia* population. However, no underlying immunosuppressive trigger has been identified and treated in this case, so there is an unquantifiable risk that the condition may recur. This dog was maintained on oral fluralaner every 3 months for routine flea and tick control, and this protocol is expected to give long term management of the *Demodex* population. There is no recurrence of clinical signs after 25 months of follow up.

Discussion

Amitraz is generally an effective medication against *Demodex*, but needs careful application and is associated with a number of potential adverse reactions. Transient sedation, as in this case, is well recognised. The sedation is caused by an alpha adrenergic agonist effect and can be reversed with 0.2 mg kg^{-1} atipamezole by intramuscular injection. Dogs can also show hypotension, bradycardia, hyperglycaemia, hypothermia and, as seen in this case, pruritus.

Fluralaner is used in this dog as a routine tick and flea control after clinical cure of the demodicosis. The fluralaner is given every 3 months by mouth, and is also available as a spot-on formulation. The use of fluralaner in normal dogs was expected to diminish the resident *Demodex* population. However, a study showed that polymerase chain reaction (PCR) analysis detected *Demodex* DNA over a 3-month period of treatment with fluralaner, suggesting that populations persist in the medium term. Further studies are needed to assess the impact of long-term fluralaner use on normal *Demodex* populations in normal dogs and on dogs that have had demodicosis in the past.

This dog first showed clinical signs of demodicosis at 9 years of age. This suggests that his immune system has maintained the resident *Demodex* population at a low subclinical level for more than 9 years and something in that balance has now changed. Potential underlying causes of adult onset generalised demodicosis include hyperadrenocorticism, multi-centric lymphoma, immunosuppressive drugs, hypothyroidism and leishmaniosis. In approximately 50% of the cases, as here, no underlying cause is identified. These dogs need ongoing monitoring for relapses of demodicosis, and may need ongoing treatment to suppress the *Demodex* population. Before the availability of isoxazolines the author attempted to take all resolved cases off medication. A good proportion of cases can continue off medication in the long term, without relapse of clinical signs or detectable *Demodex* populations.

Further reading

Fourie, J.J., Liebenberg, J.E., Horak, I.G. et al. (2015). Efficacy of orally administered fluralaner (Bravecto™) or topically applied imidacloprid/moxidectin (Advocate®) against generalized demodicosis in dogs. *Parasites and Vectors* 8: 187–197.

Zewe, C.M., Altet, L., Lam, A.T.H., and Ferrer, L. (2017). Afoxalaner and fluralaner treatment do not impact on cutaneous *Demodex* populations of healthy dogs. *Veterinary Dermatology* 28: 468–473.

History

A 7 year-old female neutered German Shepherd dog presents with slow and progressive loss of pigmentation around the face. Depigmentation of the nasal planum was first noticed 6 months ago, followed by progressive leucotrichia. White hairs are first seen at the rostral muzzle and spread in a proximal direction. The lip margins and the periocular hair become depigmented over the past 6 weeks. The dog is well, has no ocular problems and is apparently unaffected by the condition.

Questions

1. Describe the abnormalities and pertinent normal features in Figures 11.1–11.3.
2. What differential diagnoses should be considered for this presentation?
3. What tests could you perform to make the diagnosis?

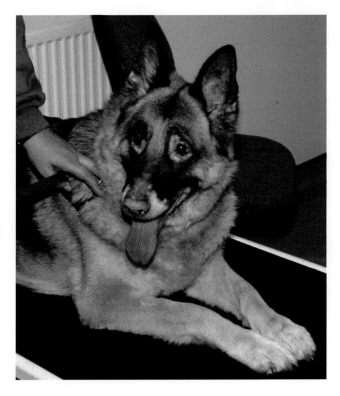

Figure 11.1

Small Animal Dermatology: What's Your Diagnosis? First Edition. Jane Coatesworth.
© 2019 John Wiley & Sons, Inc. Published 2019 by John Wiley & Sons, Inc.

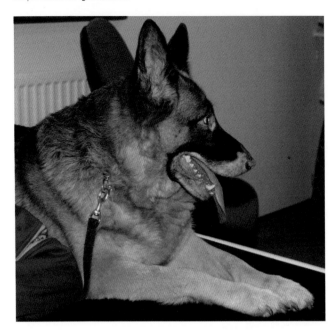

Figure 11.2

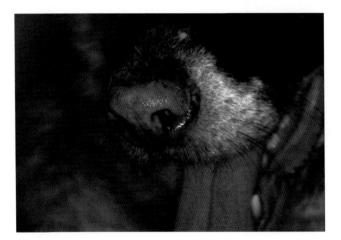

Figure 11.3

Answers

1. What the figures show

Figure 11.1 shows depigmentation of the hair around the rostral muzzle, lip margins and eyes. The leucotrichia has a bilaterally symmetrical pattern. The eyelids and nasal planum are depigmented, having previously been a solid black colour. The periocular leucotrichia forms a 6–12 mm wide band around the eyes. There are white hairs along the medial and concave aspects of both pinnae. These hairs previously had a fawn colour.

Figure 11.2 shows the right side of the dog. There is depigmentation of the hair coat and skin around the rostral muzzle and lip margins. The buccal mucosa is completely depigmented and was previously a uniform black colour. The colour of the tongue has not changed.

Figure 11.3 shows patchy depigmentation of the nasal planum. There are areas of pink, slate blue/grey and black skin. These areas represent total pigment loss, partial pigment loss and the original skin colour.

The normal cobblestone appearance of the nasal planum is retained and there is no erosion or ulceration. The hairs of the rostral muzzle are white and the vibrissae remain black.

2. **Differential diagnoses**

Given the appearance of the skin lesions the following conditions should be considered:

- Vitiligo
- Discoid lupus erythematosus (DLE). The distribution of lesions can be very similar in vitiligo and DLE, with lesions in both conditions affecting the nasal planum, rostro-dorsal muzzle, lips and peri-orbital skin. However, DLE is an inflammatory disease and often presents with swelling and crusting, and/or ulceration, in addition to the depigmentation.
- Post-inflammatory depigmentation. There is no history of trauma or inflammation. The owner has not applied any products to the affected areas and the dog is rarely off the lead, making a contact irritant or contact allergic reaction very unlikely.
- Epitheliotropic lymphoma (EL). Depigmentation at the mucocutaneous junctions can be a feature of EL. In contrast to vitiligo, EL is normally associated with variable erythema, erosion, ulceration and alopecia. The mucocutaneous junctions of the anus, prepuce and vulva are more commonly involved than in vitiligo. Most dogs with EL are, as in this case, middle-aged or older.
- Uveodermatologic syndrome. This is unlikely as the dog has no signs of ocular disease.
- Systemic lupus erythematosus. This is unlikely as the dog has no signs of systemic disease.

3. **Appropriate diagnostic tests**

Skin biopsies are taken from the margins of the affected areas. The histopathologist is looking for the absence of melanin, in an otherwise normal-appearing epidermis. Providing a biopsy sample that includes adjacent normally pigmented skin, for comparison, can make diagnosis an easier task. Skin biopsy is also helpful to rule out DLE, which is the most likely differential.

Ophthalmological examination is unremarkable. This is important to rule out uveodermatologic syndrome.

Haematology and serum biochemistry are helpful to rule out unrelated intercurrent systemic disease and systemic lupus erythematosus in this middle-aged dog.

Diagnosis

A diagnosis of vitiligo was based on the typical clinical signs, the absence of inflammation or any history of inflammation, the absence of ocular signs, the supportive histopathology and the normal architecture of the nasal planum. The gradual progression to maximal pigment loss over a 6-month period is also typical of the condition.

Treatment

There is a risk of actinic damage to the unprotected depigmented skin. A high SPF topical sun screen product is recommended, for when the affected skin is exposed to summer sunlight. Vitiligo is an immune-mediated disease, but immune-modulating treatment is not recommended. The adverse effects of treatment are likely to outweigh any benefit in this benign cosmetic condition.

Prognosis

The owner was given a very good prognosis as vitiligo is principally a cosmetic issue. Some cases remain depigmented, while others completely or partially re-pigment over an unpredictable time course. Four months later, the owner reported partial re-pigmentation of the hair around the eyes and lips and of the nasal planum.

Discussion

Vitiligo is an autoimmune disease, with auto-antibodies targeting melanocytes in the epidermis and hair follicles. The depigmentation in this case was confined to the face, but the anus, vulva, prepuce, paw pads and claws can also be affected. The condition is uncommon in the dog and rare in the cat. Clinical signs are normally seen in young adults of less than 3 years of age. The dog in this case had an unusually late age of onset. The German Shepherd dog is at increased risk of vitiligo, along with the Old English Sheepdog, Doberman Pinscher, Rottweiler, German Short Haired Pointer and Belgian Tervuren. The over-representation of certain breeds suggests a hereditary component. Male and female dogs are equally affected.

Although vitiligo is a benign condition it is important to make a definite and timely diagnosis of the cause of depigmenting changes. The clinical appearance of vitiligo can be similar to uveodermatologic syndrome and EL. Both of the latter diseases require a prompt diagnosis and treatment, to avoid poor welfare and a poor prognosis.

Non-inflammatory depigmentation restricted only to the nasal planum is seen most frequently in the yellow Labrador Retriever, Golden Retriever, Siberian Husky and Alaskan Malamute. The loss of pigment frequently only affects the area adjacent to the philtrum, and is bilaterally symmetrical. This condition, colloquially known as snow nose, usually presents with nasal depigmentation in the cold winter months and re-pigmentation in the spring and summer.

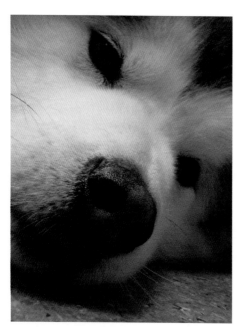

Figure 11.4 Shows a 9 year-old Siberian Husky with depigmentation of the central part of the nasal planum. There is no inflammation, erosion or ulceration and the normal architecture is unchanged. The nose re-pigments completely as the days lengthen and the ambient temperature rises in the spring, and loses pigment again as the day length decreases and the temperatures fall.

Further reading

Alhaidari, Z., Olivry, T., and Ortonne, J.-P. (1999). Melanocytogenesis and melanogenesis: genetic regulation and comparative clinical diseases. *Veterinary Dermatology* 10: 3–16.

Naughton, G.K., Mahaffey, M., and Bystryn, J.-C. (1986). Antibodies to surface antigens of pigmented cells in animals with vitiligo. In: *Proceedings of the Society of Experimental Biology and Medicine*, Blackwell Science, vol. 181, 423–426.

History

A 1 year and 8 month-old male neutered Miniature Short-haired Dachshund has a history of pruritus and of discomfort when walking. The owner noticed a rash in the right axilla 9 months ago. The affected area progressed in extent and severity despite topical zinc oxide cream and salt water bathing. The left axilla soon showed similar signs of redness and swelling. The medial aspects of the forelimbs have become involved in the past 4 months. There was some improvement with oral methylprednisolone (0.6 mg kg^{-1} on alternate days), topical chlorhexidine solution and hydrocortisone aceponate spray. The dog licks persistently at the area and is reluctant to walk. There is a low to moderate amount of scratching with the hind limbs. The dog is vaccinated and dewormed, and has monthly topical selamectin for flea control.

Questions

1. Describe the abnormalities and pertinent normal features in Figures 12.1–12.4.
2. What differential diagnoses should be considered for this presentation?
3. What tests could you perform to make the diagnosis?

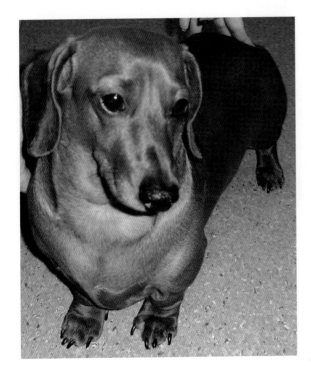

Figure 12.1

Small Animal Dermatology: What's Your Diagnosis? First Edition. Jane Coatesworth.
© 2019 John Wiley & Sons, Inc. Published 2019 by John Wiley & Sons, Inc.

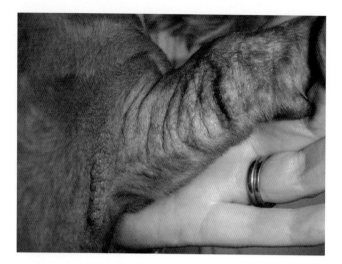

Figure 12.2

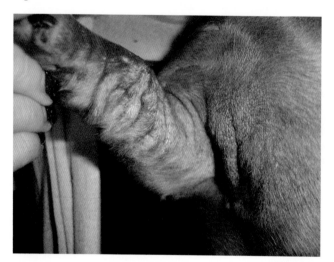

Figure 12.3

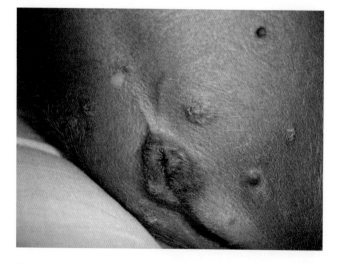

Figure 12.4

Answers

1. What the figures show

Figure 12.1 shows the dog in discomfort, and wanting to lie down. At 6.9 kg, he is significantly overweight. As soon as the owner stopped encouraging him to stand, the dog lay down with the forelimbs extended.

Figure 12.2 shows the medial aspect of the left fore limb and the adjacent body wall. There is swelling, alopecia, patchy hyperpigmentation and marked erythema of the medial forelimb. The skin is thrown into folds. The adjacent body wall is alopecic and hyperpigmented. Both areas show degrees of lichenification.

Figure 12.3 shows the medial aspect of the right fore limb and the adjacent body wall. The changes are similar to the left side. Note that the entire length of the medial fore limbs is involved.

Figure 12.4 shows the ventral abdomen. There are several large epithelial collarettes, two pustules and a large adherent crust near to the prepuce. The owner had not noticed the skin changes on the abdomen, so their duration is unknown.

2. Differential diagnoses

Given the appearance of the skin lesions the following conditions should be considered:

Primary conditions

- Atopic dermatitis and/or cutaneous adverse food reaction. These conditions present with similar clinical signs and either is likely in this young, pruritic, otherwise healthy dog with a secondary bacterial skin infection.
- Intertrigo. Friction between the leg and the body wall, when moving the fore limbs, is likely to be exacerbating the skin signs and causing discomfort and reluctance to walk. The axilla is adapted to a degree of friction by having relatively thin and glabrous skin. In this case the amount of friction is increased by skin swelling, skin folding and accumulated subcutaneous fat. Intertrigo is not the primary problem here, as skin signs extend right down the forelimbs beyond the frictional areas. Intertrigo is likely to be a contributing factor.
- Acanthosis nigricans (AN). The lesions in Figures 12.2 and 12.3 show significant inflammation. This is more suggestive of pyoderma, and/or a hypersensitivity condition, rather than of primary AN.
- Endocrinopathy, such as hypothyroidism or hyperadrenocorticism. This is unlikely but possible, given the young age of the dog. The dog is overweight and exercise intolerant, but the latter may be explained by discomfort from his skin changes.

Secondary conditions

- *Malassezia* dermatitis
- Superficial bacterial pyoderma
- Bacterial overgrowth
- Intertrigo. See previous comment

3. Appropriate diagnostic tests

Cytology. An impression smear, from the moist underside of an abdominal crust, shows degenerate neutrophils with intra and extracytoplasmic cocci. These findings are consistent with superficial bacterial pyoderma.

Acetate tape strip cytology from the axillae and medial fore limbs shows moderate to high numbers of cocci, and no *Malassezia* or inflammatory cells. These findings are consistent with a bacterial overgrowth.

Haematology and serum biochemistry are unremarkable. This dog is less than 2 years of age making endocrinopathies unlikely, but he is inactive and overweight and has a secondary skin infection.

A *food trial* is undertaken for 8 weeks using a commercial hydrolysed soya-based diet. The dog is then re-challenged with all aspects of his original diet and there is no increase in his level of pruritus. Food allergens are therefore unlikely to be contributing to his allergic skin disease.

Flea control is continued, with monthly topical selamectin. The owner is asked to spray the house with an insecticidal spray as this has not been done before. There are no other pets in the household and fleas have never been found on the dog.

Diagnosis

Canine atopic dermatitis, with secondary bacterial superficial pyoderma on the abdomen, bacterial overgrowth in the axillae and medial forelimbs, and intertrigo.

Treatment

Weight reduction to reduce the amount of subcutaneous fat, and consequent friction, between the medial forelimbs and the body wall. The dogs' bodyweight, after 2 months of dietary restriction, becomes stable at 6 kg.

Control of secondary infections. The affected skin is bathed twice weekly in a chlorhexidine based shampoo.

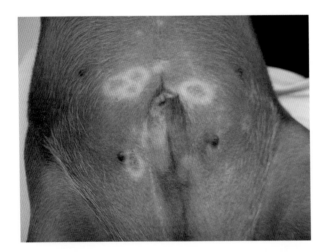

Figure 12.5 Shows the ventral abdomen 3 weeks later. There are hypopigmented macules, most with a central hyperpigmented area, at the sites of the resolved epithelial collarettes. The dog weighs 6.5 kg after 3 weeks of restricted food intake.

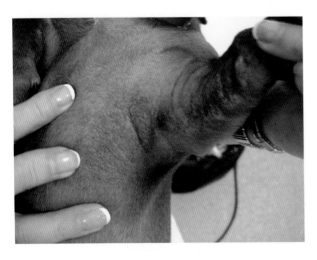

Figure 12.6 Shows the medial aspect of the left fore limb and adjacent body wall after 3 weeks of topical treatment. Much of the swelling and erythema has resolved. There is still mild erythema of the body wall, and the chronic changes of lichenification and hyperpigmentation.

Treatment of atopic dermatitis. Once the secondary bacterial infection and bacterial overgrowth has resolved and the dog has lost weight, there is only a mildly increased degree of pruritus above that of a normal dog. Topical hydrocortisone aceponate spray is used once every week on pruritic and potentially pruritic areas of skin. The pruritic areas are initially the axillae and groin, but later also include the interdigital spaces of the front paws. After 3 months of treatment the dog is comfortable, and has a low and stable level of pruritus. Allergen specific immunotherapy is discussed with the owner as a possible future treatment option should the clinical signs become more apparent.

Prognosis

The prognosis is good if the underlying disease, potential secondary infections and the body weight are all kept under control.

Discussion

Primary AN is a rare disease that is seen in Dachshunds. The breed specificity suggests that a genetic contribution is likely, but the mode of inheritance has not been established. The first clinical signs can be seen from 3 months of age and signs are usually apparent at less than 2 years of age. Males and females are equally affected. Some dermatologists have termed the post-inflammatory hyperpigmentation of the axillae and groin as secondary AN. The author prefers to use the term AN only for the Dachshund specific genodermatosis.

Secondary AN is far more commonly encountered than primary AN and occurs in a variety of breeds including the Dachshund. The focal inflammation of the axillae, and subsequent hyperpigmentation, can have a variety of underlying causes. Endocrinopathies, such as hypothyroidism and hyperadrenocorticism, can predispose to hyperpigmentation, secondary infection and weight gain. These conditions are mostly seen in middle-aged dogs. Allergic skin disease such as the atopic dermatitis in this case, but also cutaneous adverse food reaction and flea bite hypersensitivity, can cause ongoing inflammation and pruritus of the axillary skin and predispose to secondary infections. Clinical signs of atopic dermatitis tend to first occur in young dogs, but fleas and food can induce hypersensitivity at any age.

The diagnosis of atopic dermatitis is a clinical diagnosis made by exclusion. Intradermal skin testing or IgE serology could be performed in this case at a later date, if the clinical signs progress. These tests cannot differentiate atopic from non-atopic dogs. They are useful to guide the formulation of an immunotherapy vaccine, or to guide the avoidance of certain allergens, for dogs that are already known to be atopic.

The dog has a bacterial superficial pyoderma on the abdomen, but only in a restricted area. Topical antimicrobial therapy is used rather than systemic antibiotics. Systemic antibiotics may be appropriate if topical therapy is unsuccessful and the pyoderma is progressive. Clindamycin would be an option as the dog has not had antibiotics before. Clindamycin can be given once daily and the owner finds it difficult to administer tablets. Systemic antibiotics are not indicated for bacterial overgrowth and it is best treated with topical antimicrobial therapy.

Hydrocortisone aceponate has a potent anti-inflammatory and anti-pruritic action in the skin. This diester formulation is many times more potent than hydrocortisone. It is lipophilic and has good penetration into the skin. Hydrocortisone aceponate is at least as effective as topical dexamethasone or betamethasone. It is broken down in the dermis and there is minimal systemic absorption. Hydrocortisone aceponate is available as a 0.0584% spray formulation, in a volatile liquid carrier. The spray distributes the product onto the skin in a fine layer and is very useful for localised inflammatory lesions, as in this case. Hydrocortisone aceponate is best applied on an intermittent basis when used in the long term, for example on 1 or 2 days each week. The product has been used on a proactive long term basis, on two consecutive days each week, in dogs with atopic dermatitis to give extended periods of remission between flares of the disease. Frequent long term use is not recommended and can lead to atrophic skin changes and suppression of the hypothalamus pituitary axis. The data sheet recommends daily application for up to seven consecutive days, and only spraying up to one-third of the skin surface area each day. It is important to avoid any spray from contacting the eyes. The product is flammable in both liquid and vapour form.

Further reading

Lourenço, A.M., Schmidt, V., São Braz, B. et al. (2016). Efficacy of proactive long-term maintenance therapy of canine atopic dermatitis with 0.0584% hydrocortisone aceponate spray: a double-blind placebo controlled pilot study. *Veterinary Dermatology* 27: 88–92.

History

A 6 year-old female neutered Bernese Mountain dog presents as an ophthalmological emergency with bilateral uveitis and secondary glaucoma in the right eye. Two years ago, there was an episode of bilateral ocular pain and inflammation, along with crusting and inflammation around the eyes, lips and nose. This resolves, after a course of topical glucocorticoids and systemic antibiotics, leaving depigmentation of the skin and hair coat around the eyes. The leucotrichia progresses steadily, over the past 2 years, to involve the whole body. The brown areas of hair coat, on the legs, are the last to be affected. Three weeks ago, the dog again shows bilateral ocular pain and inflammation, this improves with topical anti-inflammatories but glaucoma subsequently develops in the right eye. The dog is regularly dewormed and vaccinated and is receiving daily non-steroidal anti-inflammatory medication (meloxicam) for degenerative joint disease. Tibial plateau levelling osteotomy surgery was performed on the left stifle 1 year ago.

Questions

1. Describe the abnormalities and pertinent normal features in Figures 13.1–13.6.
2. What differential diagnoses should be considered for this presentation?
3. What tests could you perform to make the diagnosis?

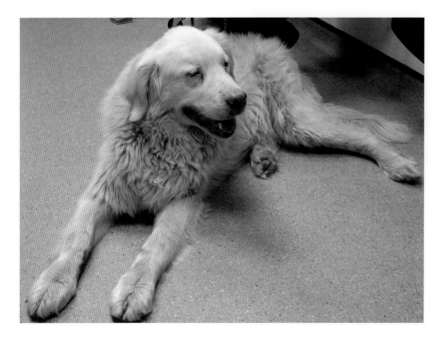

Figure 13.1

Small Animal Dermatology: What's Your Diagnosis? First Edition. Jane Coatesworth.
© 2019 John Wiley & Sons, Inc. Published 2019 by John Wiley & Sons, Inc.

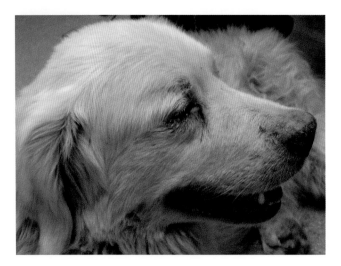

Figure 13.2

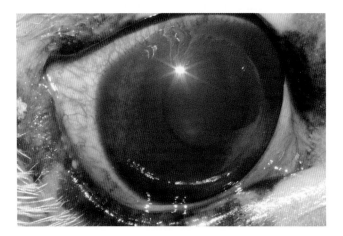

Figure 13.3

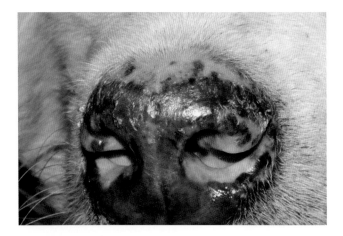

Figure 13.4

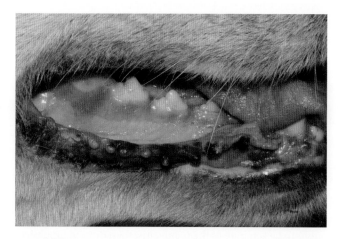

Figure 13.5

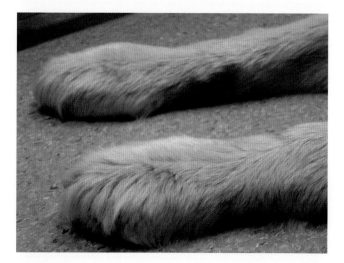

Figure 13.6

Answers

1. What the figures show

Figure 13.1 shows the dog lying on the floor. There is almost total loss of hair coat pigmentation in comparison to the appearance of a normal tri-coloured Bernese Mountain dog. The extent and severity of leucotrichia has progressed over the past 2 years, starting around the eyes at 4 years of age. The dog is panting despite the moderate ambient temperature suggesting anxiety or pain. There is persistent bilateral blepharospasm, suggesting photophobia and/or ocular pain.

Figure 13.2 shows the right side of the head. There is inflammation around the eyes and lips, and at the rostro-dorsal muzzle. The dog is panting and has blepharospasm. Traces of yellow fluorescein dye are visible on the coat around the eye, after assessing the cornea for ulceration.

Figure 13.3 shows the right eye. There is extensive depigmentation, and some swelling and erythema of the lids. The conjunctiva, overlying the sclera, is markedly hyperaemic and has congested blood vessels. There is diffuse corneal oedema and intraocular inflammation (aqueous flare). Fundoscopy shows multifocal areas of depigmentation in the non-tapetal area of the retina, but no retinal detachment.

Figure 13.4 shows the nasal planum. There is complete depigmentation of the nostrils and the dorsal aspect of the nasal planum. There is partial depigmentation over most of the nasal planum giving a grey colour. The normal 'cobblestone' appearance is lost and there is some adherent crust over the dorsal third of the nasal planum. A few small areas of the original black nasal colour are retained laterally.

Figure 13.5 shows the right side of the mouth. There is partial patchy depigmentation of the lip margins. The lip margins are erythematous and swollen, with adherent overlying crust at the commissures. The pattern is bilaterally symmetrical.

Figure 13.6 shows extensive depigmentation of the distal forelimbs. Discrete patches of brown hair remain at the medial and lateral metacarpal areas.

2. **Differential diagnoses**

Given the appearance of the skin and eye lesions the following conditions should be considered:

- Uveodermatologic syndrome (UDS) is the only likely cause here, given the history and clinical signs of concurrent inflammation and extensive depigmentation affecting both the eyes and the skin.
- If the depigmenting skin lesions were thought to be separate to the panuveitis, then discoid lupus erythematosus, vitiligo and epitheliotropic lymphoma would also be considered. Erosion and ulceration of the nasal planum can occur with uveodermatologic syndrome. Differentials for this would include leishmaniosis, localised pemphigus foliaceus and discoid lupus erythematosus.

3. **Appropriate diagnostic tests**

Ophthalmological examination is very important, as the condition is painful and potentially blinding. There is a mucopurulent discharge in both eyes. Both the palpebral and bulbar conjunctivae are markedly hyperaemic. Some deep peri-limbal hyperaemia is also present. There is diffuse corneal oedema in both eyes, and marked intraocular inflammation (aqueous flare). The intraocular pressures are 19 mmHg in the right eye and 12 mmHg in the left eye (normal intraocular pressure 10–20 mmHg). The pressure in the right eye spikes at 29 mmHg during hospitalisation. The pressure in the left eye is low due to the uveitis. The pressure in the right eye is relatively high despite the concurrent uveitis and suggestive of glaucoma. Secondary glaucoma is a common complication of severe intraocular inflammation.

Haematology and serum biochemistry results are all within normal limits. These values provide a useful reference baseline before starting immunosuppressive therapy.

Skin biopsies can be useful in early cases with less pathognomic clinical signs. Histopathology typically shows a band of inflammatory cells lying in the superficial dermis, just underneath the junction with the epidermis. Uveodermatologic syndrome needs to be differentiated from other diseases that show this lichenoid band, such as discoid lupus erythematosus.

Brain auditory evoked response *(BAER) testing* shows normal peripheral thresholds in both ears, consistent with normal hearing. Functioning melanocytes, in the cochlea of the inner ear, are important for normal hearing. Deafness can be a feature of the analogous Vogt–Koyanagi–Harada syndrome in people. Deafness is not reported in uveodermatologic syndrome in the dog, but is rarely assessed.

Diagnosis

Uveodermatologic syndrome (UDS).

Treatment

The dog is started on an immunosuppressive dose (50 mg m^{-2}) of both oral prednisolone and azathioprine. Meloxicam is discontinued. She is kept in the hospital for intensive topical treatment of both eyes, with 1% prednisolone acetate and 20 mg ml^{-1} dorzolamide hydrochloride, and to monitor the intraocular pressures. After 4 days of treatment and monitoring, the dog is returned to the owners' care with continued systemic prednisolone and azathioprine and with topical prednisolone drops to apply to both eyes every 4 hours. The intraocular pressures are 7 mmHg in both eyes.

Haematology results show neutrophilia and eosinopenia. The alkaline phosphatase (ALP), alanine aminotransferase (ALT), bile acids, total bilirubin and cholesterol values are all significantly elevated.

Prognosis

The prognosis is guarded. The severe panuveitis, which is often present in this condition, can be recurrent and painful and can lead to blindness.

Further treatment and outcome

Ten days later, examination shows no evidence of active intraocular inflammation. The intraocular pressures are 24 and 11 mmHg in the right and left eye, respectively. The dog can see, the eyes appear to be comfortable and the panting has stopped. There appears to be a moderate amount of joint stiffness in the limbs.

Haematology results show a mild regenerative anaemia and a neutrophilia. The ALP, ALT, bile acids, total bilirubin and cholesterol values are all persistently elevated. An ultrasound scan of the abdomen shows an enlarged liver with rounded margins and a slightly patchy echotexture.

Anaemia is a possible adverse drug effect of azathioprine although the drug-related anaemia, due to bone marrow suppression, is normally non-regenerative and accompanied by thrombocytopenia and neutropenia. This dog has no thrombocytopenia and a neutropenia could be masked by the neutrophilia associated with corticosteroid administration. The regenerative anaemia seen here could be associated with glucocorticoid induced gastrointestinal ulceration and bleeding. The high serum biochemistry values may be associated with azathioprine hepatotoxicosis, or with the effects of the exogenous glucocorticoids.

Azathioprine is discontinued, and the dose of systemic prednisolone is halved to 25 mg m^{-2} q 24 hours. Omeprazole (1 mg kg^{-1} q 24 hours), which inhibits gastric acid secretion, is started as a gastroprotectant. S-adenosyl-L-methionine (SAM-e) supplementation is started as a hepatoprotectant (450 mg q 24 hours, given 1 hour before food) and ciclosporin (5 mg kg^{-1} q 24 hours) as an alternative immuno-modulating drug. Topical prednisolone is continued every 4 hours in both eyes, and topical dorzolamide hydrochloride, a carbonic anhydrase inhibitor, is restarted every 8 hours in the right eye.

Ten days later, the dog is polydypsic, polyuric and slightly lethargic. She has difficulty rising from recumbency and is reluctant to walk on slippery floors. The abdomen is distended, but not uncomfortable on palpation. Ocular examination shows no evidence of intraocular inflammation. The intraocular pressures are 6 mmHg in both eyes. There is crepitus, stiffness and pain in a variety of joints involving all four limbs. There are no proprioceptive deficits or palpable joint effusions. The left hind limb is significantly abducted when walking. The dog is given tramadol but becomes recumbent and unable to rise. The owners elect to have the dog euthanised. The marked and rapid deterioration in limb function was thought to be related to the absence of meloxicam, the known intercurrent degenerative joint disease and to corticosteroid or ciclosporin induced muscle weakness.

Discussion

UDS is sometimes described as Vogt–Koyanagi–Harada-like syndrome, to signal similarity to a human condition described by a Swiss and two Japanese ophthalmologists. In contrast to the human condition, the dog is thought to rarely have a meningoencephalitis component to the disease, although this aspect may be poorly recognised.

The syndrome is an immune-mediated disease, with antibodies attacking melanocytes in both the skin and the eye. The depigmentation of the skin and hair coat is usually seen, in a symmetrical pattern, around the mucocutaneous junctions. The lips, periocular and perinasal skin are commonly involved. Depigmentation started in these areas in this case, then progressed to involve most of the body. Such extensive depigmentation is unusual, but this case had probably had active disease for at least 2 years. Similar cases, with generalised depigmentation, have been reported in a Shetland Sheepdog and a Dachshund. Other cases, but with only localised depigmentation, have been reported in the Bernese Mountain dog.

Although the skin and hair coat changes are visually striking, they are largely cosmetic and urgent treatment needs to focus on the inflammatory changes in the eyes. The eyes can be affected by bilateral anterior uveitis or panuveitis, depigmentation of the iris or choroid, retinal detachment and blindness. Secondary changes may include cataracts, adhesions between the iris and the lens (posterior synechiae) and, as in this case, glaucoma.

UDS was first reported in Japan in 1977, and in the UK in 1987. The Japanese Akita is the most commonly reported breed, suggesting a hereditary component in this breed. Young adult dogs, as in this 4 year-old, are most commonly affected. There is no sex predilection.

Immunosuppressive treatment is associated with a fairly high incidence of adverse drug reactions. Regular blood tests and clinical assessments are important to monitor for the potential adverse effects of medication. The marked changes in serum biochemistry values seen in this case are probably due to hepatopathy, caused by the combination of azathioprine and corticosteroids. In one study the observed frequency of azathioprine associated hepatotoxicosis, as defined by a greater than two-fold increase in ALT activity, was 15%. Within this 15% many cases showed no clinical signs. The ALT activity in this case had a greater than 10-fold increase. The elevated ALP levels are likely due to a combination of steroid induced elevation and hepatopathy.

Cytotoxic drugs, such as azathioprine, are often dosed on a metre squared basis. This gives a more accurate dose for the larger and smaller dogs. For example, this dog weighs 50 kg. The daily dose of azathioprine is 68.5 mg at 50 mg m^{-2} and 100 mg at 2 mg kg^{-1}, representing a significant difference.

Azathioprine hepatotoxicosis is exacerbated experimentally by glutathione depletion. SAM-e supplementation acts as a glutathione precursor and is a logical, but unproven, treatment option for this condition in the dog. Azathioprine is converted, in the body, to the active form 6-mercaptopurine. The capacity to convert 6-mercaptopurine to inactive metabolites varies between individual dogs and has a genetic basis. Dogs with a limited ability to denature 6-mercaptopurine are more likely to be at risk of drug induced bone marrow suppression.

Further reading

Asakura, S., Takahashi, K., and Onishi, T. (1977). Vogt-Koyanagi-Harada syndrome (uveitis diffusa acuta) in the dog. *Journal of the Veterinary Medicine (Japan)* 673: 445–455.

Cottrell, B.D. and Barnett, K.C. (1987). Harada's disease in the Japanese Akita. *Journal of Small Animal Practice* 28: 517–521.

Hendrix, D. (2013). Chapter 20: diseases and surgery of the canine anterior uvea. In: *Veterinary Ophthalmology*, 5e (ed. K.N. Gelatt, B.C. Gilger and T.J. Kern), 1165–1166. Oxford, UK: Wiley-Blackwell.

Wallisch, K. and Trepanier, L.A. (2015). Incidence, timing, and risk factors of azathioprine hepatotoxicosis in dogs. *Journal of Veterinary Internal Medicine* 29: 513–518.

History

A 10 year-old male entire Papillon is presented with a history of colour change on the nose. The dog previously had an entirely black nose. The owners have noticed the loss of black coloration, in patches, over the past 2 months. The dog is bright and well, and shows no signs of discomfort or irritation from the skin.

Questions

1. Describe the abnormalities and pertinent normal features in Figures 14.1 and 14.2.
2. What differential diagnoses should be considered for this presentation?
3. What tests could you perform to make the diagnosis?

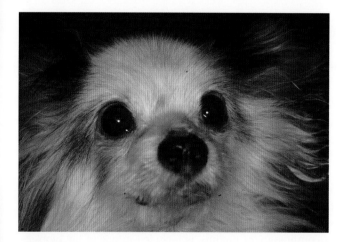

Figure 14.1

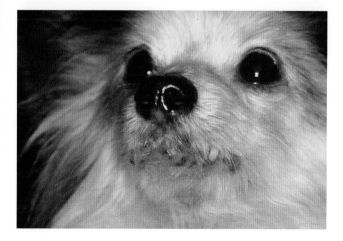

Figure 14.2

Small Animal Dermatology: What's Your Diagnosis? First Edition. Jane Coatesworth.
© 2019 John Wiley & Sons, Inc. Published 2019 by John Wiley & Sons, Inc.

Answers

1. What the figures show

Figure 14.1 shows the face and is focussed on the eyes. There is depigmentation, mild swelling and erythema of the upper and lower eyelids. The conjunctivae are inflamed and there is an overflow of tears causing skin wetness below the eyes.

Figure 14.2 shows the face and is focussed on the rostral muzzle. There is a patch of depigmentation at the base of the philtrum and areas of partial depigmentation elsewhere on the nasal planum. The nasal planum is somewhat swollen and has lost the normal cobblestone surface texture. There is almost total depigmentation and mild swelling of the lip margins. A 3-mm diameter erythematous plaque is present at the left commissure of the lips.

2. Differential diagnoses

Given the appearance of the skin lesions the following conditions should be considered:

- Epitheliotropic lymphoma (EL)
- Vitiligo

These conditions can have a similar appearance, although the mucocutaneous form of EL usually presents with inflammation as well as depigmentation. Vitiligo is a benign cosmetic disease and does not have visible inflammation or changes of architecture. Biopsy is essential to make a diagnosis in this older dog.

3. Appropriate diagnostic tests

Physical examination shows that the lesions are restricted to the face. There is no peripheral lymphadenopathy, or involvement of other areas of skin or mucous membranes.

Routine *haematology and serum biochemistry* results are unremarkable in this older dog. The blood results give useful pre-anaesthetic information, give a baseline for future monitoring while on treatment and rule out a number of inter-current conditions.

Skin biopsies. Full thickness 6-mm diameter punch biopsies are taken from the lip margin and the nasal planum. Visually affected skin is selected, including some adjacent skin with normal pigmentation. The entire 3-mm plaque, at the left commissure of the lips, is included in one of the biopsies. Histopathology shows diffuse infiltration of the epidermis, hair follicles, sweat and sebaceous glands, by small lymphoid cells. This pattern is characteristic of EL.

Cytology can be helpful to demonstrate the presence of a round cell tumour when there are ulcerated or solid lesions to sample. Cytology was not a realistic option in this case as the skin surface was intact and the single small plaque was only just raised above the skin surface. Although cytology can be used to diagnose some round cell tumours, they often need further characterisation by biopsy and histopathology. The round cell tumour family includes cutaneous and non-cutaneous lymphoma, mast cell tumour, histiocytoma, Merkel cell tumour, melanoma and transmissible venereal tumour.

Diagnosis

EL. The diagnosis was based on the suggestive history and clinical signs, and confirmed by histopathology.

Treatment

The owner declined any treatment and decided that the dog would be put to sleep when adverse effects of the disease became apparent. Treatment is aimed at improving the quality of life and is currently not curative.

Prognosis

The prognosis is poor. Most dogs with EL are euthanised months, rather than years, after diagnosis. This is partly because the condition is seldom recognised in the early stages and tends to be advanced by the time a diagnosis is made. Treatment improves quality of life but generally has little impact on extending lifespan. EL is a progressive disease. The condition can become generalised, with extension to the lymph nodes and other organs, but many dogs are euthanised before this stage.

Final outcome

Two months later the owner notices excess scale throughout the coat and generalised reddening of the skin. The dog has a bright demeanour and no apparent skin discomfort.

Four months later, the dog is euthanised at the owner's request. There has been increasing pruritus, characterised by generalised licking and scratching. The dog has developed peripheral lymphadenopathy, and has become lethargic and miserable.

Discussion

EL occurs when a T memory lymphocyte undergoes neoplastic transformation and subsequent clonal proliferation. The population of neoplastic lymphocytes then migrates to and infiltrates into the superficial skin. The cause of the neoplasia is not understood. A history of chronic inflammatory skin disease may be a predisposing factor, although there was no such history in this case. The mean age at diagnosis is 8.6 years. This number may be significantly higher than the age of onset, as EL is often mistakenly assumed to be an inflammatory skin condition and is consequently not biopsied early in the course of disease. The Cocker Spaniel and Boxer breeds appear to be predisposed. There is no sex predisposition.

The clinical signs of EL are very variable, and can mimic a range of other skin diseases. There can be plaques and nodules, erythema and scaling, alopecia and erosion and, as in this case, depigmentation of the skin and mucous membranes. Intense erythema and ulceration of the oral mucosa can be a feature. The degree of pruritus varies from nothing to significant. Scaling and diffuse redness of the haired skin often precedes the appearance of plaques and nodules, and is most often seen over the torso and head.

The diagnosis in this case was clear from the compatible history, clinical signs and histopathology. When the diagnosis is less clear immunophenotyping can be helpful, either by flow cytometry or by immuno-histochemistry. Immunophenotyping can differentiate between B and T lymphocytes, give cell sizes and indicate the level of cell maturity. PCR for antigen receptor rearrangements (PARR) is a PCR assay of cell DNA. PARR can be useful in selected cases to understanding the clonality of a population of infiltrating lymphocytes. EL has a monoclonal population, while the infiltration of reactive lymphocytes in inflammatory skin disease will be polyclonal. PARR can give false positive and false negative results and needs careful interpretation.

The most helpful treatment for EL, with current knowledge, is lomustine (also known as CCNU). This drug is an alkylating agent. It works by attaching an alkyl group to DNA, and causing DNA damage in body cells that are dividing and multiplying. The target tumour population is compromised by the drug, but other rapidly dividing cells in the body are also susceptible to damage. Adverse effects include bone marrow suppression, which can manifest as thrombocytopenia, anaemia and/or leukopenia. Gastrointestinal signs include vomiting, diarrhoea and anorexia. Hepatic and renal toxicity are uncommon but can be severe. Lomustine is given by mouth, typically every 3–8 weeks for four cycles. The dog's wellbeing and blood parameters are assessed prior to each dose, allowing the treatment to be tailored to the individual response. The response rate to lomustine is generally high, at around 80%. However, the duration of the response is generally short (3–4 months), before further progression of the disease is apparent.

Anti-inflammatory doses of prednisolone can be helpful to reduce the associated inflammation and pruritus, and to improve quality of life. Prednisolone can be given alone, or in combination with lomustine.

Further reading

Fontaine, J., Bovens, C., Bettenay, S., and Mueller, R.S. (2008). Canine cutaneous epitheliotropic T-cell lymphoma: a review. *Veterinary and Comparative Oncology* 7: 1–14.

Risbon, R.E., Lorimier, L.P., Skorupski, K. et al. (2006). Response of canine cutaneous epitheliotropic lymphoma to lomustine (CCNU): a retrospective study of 46 cases (1999–2004). *Journal of Veterinary Internal Medicine* 20: 1389–1397.

Williams, L.E., Rassnick, K.M., Power, H.T. et al. (2006). CCNU in the treatment of canine epitheliotropic lymphoma. *Journal of Veterinary Internal Medicine* 20: 136–143.

Pruritus

Itchy dogs and cats can cause variable degrees of skin damage through self-trauma, although owners are not always aware of the excessive scratching and licking. Pruritic behaviour can result in excoriation, ulceration and erosion of the skin, with subsequent exudation and even bleeding. The hair shafts can be fractured or whole hairs can be pulled out, resulting in hypotrichosis or alopecia. Abrasion of the skin contributes to reduced barrier function and secondary bacterial infections. Cats are particularly able to cause significant skin damage in a short period of time, especially if the hind claws are sharp.

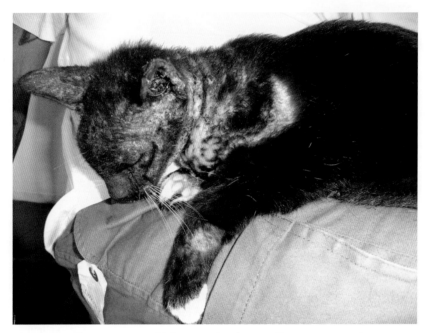

Figure C.1   Shows a 10 year-old domestic shorthair cat. There is severe and widespread self-inflicted skin trauma of the head, neck, shoulders and forelimbs. The affected skin is abraded by licking and by scratching with the hind legs. The rest of the body is unaffected and has a normal hair coat. This case was lost to follow-up.

Simple interventions, such as cutting the claws short and flat or fitting soft plastic nail covers, can reduce the potential for self-trauma. The use of Elizabethan collars and protective clothing needs assessment of the balance of risk to benefit for the individual animal. Physically preventing an animal from scratching may be justified in the short term, but is not a long term solution and may contribute to an increased level of stress and a reduced level of welfare.

Small Animal Dermatology: What's Your Diagnosis? First Edition. Jane Coatesworth.
© 2019 John Wiley & Sons, Inc. Published 2019 by John Wiley & Sons, Inc.

It can be helpful to ask specific questions about itch. The question 'Is he/she itchy?' will be answered depending on the owners' assessment of what compromises itch. Foot washing may be interpreted as being clean, scooting on the perineum as only associated with impaction of the anal sacs and dragging the ventrum along the carpet as a party trick. Some owners associate itch only with scratching behaviour using a hind limb. Owners may not associate itch with rubbing, chewing, scooting, pawing, gnawing, nibbling, licking or head shaking, and so may not share this valuable information unless specifically asked.

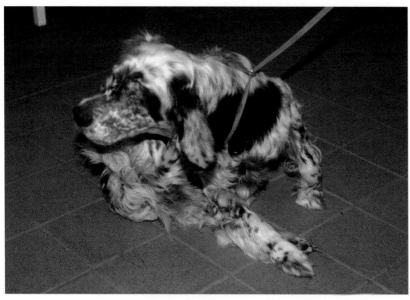

Figure C.2 Shows a young female English Setter. The dog is using the right hind leg to scratch at the right neck. This type of behaviour is widely understood by owners to mean that the dog is itchy and help is sought for these dogs in a timely manner. Other types of pruritic behaviour may not be so readily associated with itch. This dog shows widespread erythema and has atopic dermatitis.

Scratching is a reflex response to itch. The next time you have a sensation of itch try to be aware of it, but to not make any response to the sensation. It requires a strong conscious effort to disassociate the perception of itch from the response to itch. Animals that have been reprimanded for showing pruritic behaviour will often find themselves in conflict, which may increase their stress levels. These animals may try to alleviate the pruritus when they are not being observed. Some animals will show a repetitive oral behaviour, such as foot licking, when stressed. This type of behaviour is thought to be a strategy for mitigating stress by stimulating the release of endogenous opioids. Contemporary pets tend to live in human environments and by human rules, and may have limited options for balancing their needs. Psychological stress is a factor in the exacerbation of some skin diseases in people and this may also apply to dogs and cats.

The physical examination of a pruritic patient can reveal evidence of itchy behaviour. There may be hair under the gum margins, especially around the canine teeth. Frequent licking can result in reddish brown staining of a pale coloured hair coat due to the porphyrins found in saliva. Tape strips may reveal the oral commensal bacteria *Simonsiella* on the skin where animals have been licking. Areas of traumatised and broken hairs have a spiky stubbly texture when we run our hands over the hair coat.

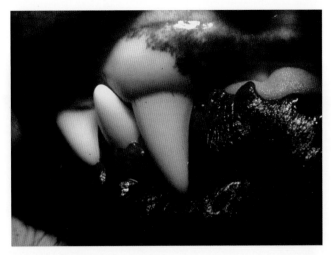

Figure C.3 Shows the left canine tooth of a young black Labrador Retriever with atopic dermatitis. There are a number of hairs trapped under the gum margin at the base of the upper canine tooth. The dog frequently nibbles and gnaws down the front limbs and in the antecubital fossae.

The most common causes of pruritus are parasites, infections and/or allergic skin disease. These are 'the big three' and they should be considered in the differential diagnosis of any case involving pruritus.

Tactful enquiries about skin lesions in owners can give helpful clues in the diagnosis of a pruritic pet. *Sarcoptes* and *Cheyletiella* mites, fleas and dermatophytes can all cause zoonotic disease in owners that have close contact with their pets or share the same environments.

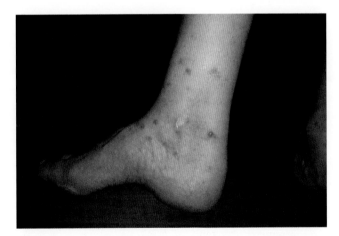

Figure C.4 Shows the lower right leg of a cat owner. There are multiple erythematous and pruritic papules resulting from flea bites. Fleas and flea dirt were not found on the indoor/outdoor cat probably due to meticulous grooming behaviour, but fleas were found in the house.

The concept of a pruritic threshold is useful in understanding the specific trigger factors and therapeutic needs of an individual patient. Each individual is thought to have a level or threshold of pruritus above which the animal is itchy. The pruritic threshold varies between individuals and may move up or down for an individual over time. In some individuals the uncomplicated primary disease, such as atopic dermatitis, may be significant enough to put them above their pruritic threshold. Factors that contribute to itch are cumulative. For example, an allergic dog may not exceed its pruritic threshold, but the same dog with a superficial pyoderma may exceed threshold and be pruritic. Additional factors, such as a hot day and a flea burden, can increase the degree of pruritus. The aim of medication and environmental modification is to address the various factors that contribute to the pruritus and to have the patient at or just below their pruritic threshold. A patient with a chronic pruritic disease that never shows any pruritic behaviour may be receiving an unnecessary amount of medication.

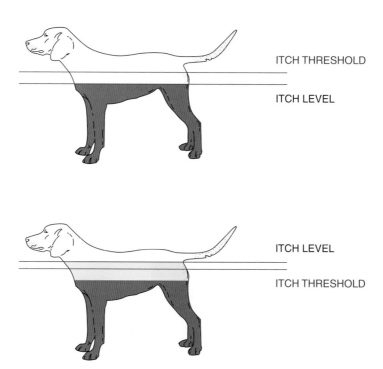

Figure C.5 Is a diagram showing the concept of a pruritic threshold. The various factors that contribute to pruritus add together. As more factors accrue, the pruritic threshold is more likely to be exceeded and the animal will become pruritic. In the top diagram, the itch level is below the itch threshold and the dog is not itchy; for example, uncomplicated atopic dermatitis. In the lower diagram, the itch level is above the itch threshold and the dog is itchy; for example, atopic dermatitis (purple contribution to itch) plus a bacterial superficial pyoderma (yellow contribution to itch).

History

A 15 month-old male neutered West Highland White Terrier presents with a history of pruritus. The dog is vaccinated and dewormed and has regular flea control. He eats a commercial complete lamb and rice-based dry diet with an occasional treat of cheese. The owners are not affected by any skin problems and there are no other animals in the household. At 6 months of age, the dog has mild superficial bacterial pyoderma on the ventral abdomen. This clears after bathing the affected area in antimicrobial shampoo. At 8 months of age, the dog starts to lick and chew at the dorsal aspects of the fore limbs, and at the dorsal and palmar aspects of the front paws. Skin scrapes from the legs and feet do not reveal any ectoparasites. The diet is changed for an 8-week period to a commercial complete fish and potato-based diet. There is no overall change in the level of pruritus, although it waxes and wanes. A further 8 weeks on, a commercial hydrolysed soy diet also results in no overall change in the level of itch. The owner assesses the itch score to be 7/10, and feels that the dog is less active and has a depressed demeanour.

Questions

1. Describe the abnormalities and pertinent normal features in Figures 15.1–15.4.
2. What differential diagnoses should be considered for this presentation?
3. What tests could you perform to make the diagnosis?

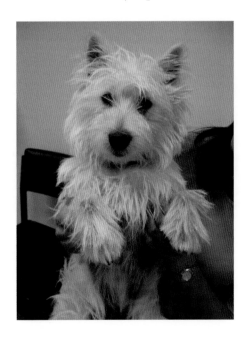

Figure 15.1

Small Animal Dermatology: What's Your Diagnosis? First Edition. Jane Coatesworth.
© 2019 John Wiley & Sons, Inc. Published 2019 by John Wiley & Sons, Inc.

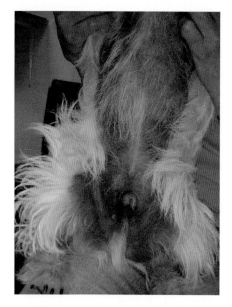

Figure 15.2

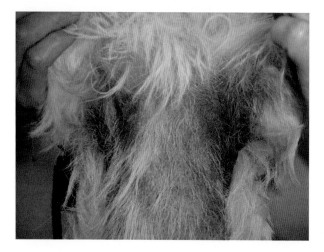

Figure 15.3

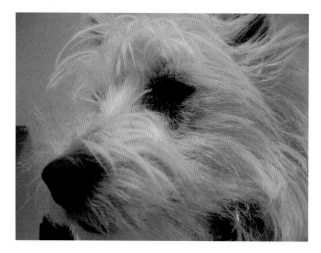

Figure 15.4

Answers

1. **What the figures show**

Figure 15.1 shows a front view of the dog. There is hypotrichosis and erythema over the dorsal aspect of the fore limbs.

Figure 15.2 shows the ventral chest, ventral abdomen, groin and hind legs. There is extensive patchy erythema, alopecia and hyperpigmentation. The skin is thickened and lichenified.

Figure 15.3 shows the ventral chest and axillae. There is moderate erythema and mild hyperpigmentation of the ventral chest, and marked hyperpigmentation and lichenification of the axillae.

Figure 15.4 shows the left face. There is marked hyperpigmentation of the periocular skin and yellow/brown staining of the periocular hair. The skin at and ventral to the medial canthus is wet and hypotrichotic. The skin changes are similar on the right periocular area.

2. **Differential diagnoses**

Given the appearance of the skin lesions the following conditions should be considered:

Parasites
- Demodicosis
- Sarcoptic mange

Infections
- Bacterial superficial pyoderma (there are no focal lesions suggestive of this)
- *Malassezia* dermatitis

Hypersensitivity conditions
- Atopic dermatitis
- Flea bite hypersensitivity
- Cutaneous adverse food reaction. This has been ruled out by the lack of improvement in clinical signs during two dietary trials, with good owner compliance

3. **Appropriate diagnostic tests**

Skin scrapes are repeated to rule out generalised demodicosis in this young dog. The dog is receiving regular topical selamectin as flea control. This product would also control *Sarcoptes* mites.

Hair plucks from around the eyes show numerous hairs with fractured shafts, suggestive of self-trauma and pruritus in this area. No *Demodex* mites are found.

Acetate strip cytology from the axillae, interdigital spaces and groin do not show any cocci, *Malassezia* or inflammatory cells. There are numerous *Simonsiella* and *Malassezia* on tape strips from the groin, suggesting licking or chewing behaviour in this area that has not been seen by the owner. Tape strips from the periocular skin show high numbers of cocci and rods, and no inflammatory cells.

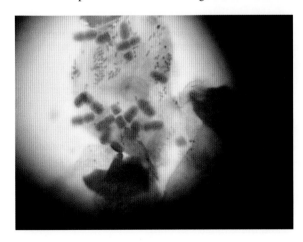

Figure 15.5 Shows a magnified area of an acetate tape strip, taken from the abdominal skin and stained with Rapi-Diff. The image is taken through the microscope. The arrangement of 'stacked' parallel rods is characteristic of *Simonsiella*. This Gram-negative bacteria is part of the normal oral flora and finding it on tape strips is suggestive of licking and gnawing behaviour. There are also numerous *Malassezia*, especially in the top half of the image. The *Malassezia* are much smaller than the *Simonsiella* aggregates. *Simonsiella* are usually seen attached to a large angular epithelial cell, as in this image.

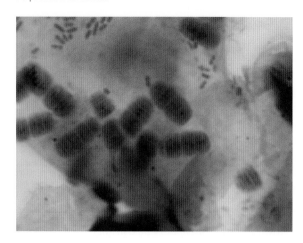

Figure 15.6 Shows an enlarged image of a few of the *Simonsiella* aggregates. The rods, lying in parallel, can be seen more clearly.

Intradermal testing and *IgE serology* show no positive results. A small proportion of dogs, with a clinical diagnosis of atopic dermatitis made by exclusion, do not have positive results on intradermal or serological testing. These dogs are described as having atopic-like dermatitis and cannot benefit from allergen specific immunotherapy or allergen avoidance. Dogs in this group may go on to develop an IgE response to allergens, may be allergic to something we are not testing for or may have an alternative disease mechanism that is not mediated by IgE. Approximately 20% of people with atopic dermatitis have the 'intrinsic' form and have normal levels of IgE.

Diagnosis

Atopic-like dermatitis with bacterial overgrowth around the eyes and *Malassezia* overgrowth in the groin.

Treatment

The owner is shown how to wash the periocular skin with dilute povidone iodine solution and asked to wash the area twice daily for 10 days to reduce the bacterial overgrowth. A 0.3% chlorhexidine/TrizEDTA gel is used once daily, on the abdominal skin, to reduce the *Malassezia* overgrowth. Ciclosporin, at $5 \, \mathrm{mg\,kg^{-1}}$ once daily, is started to try to address the underlying inflammatory skin disease. Regular flea control is continued.

Four weeks later there is a dramatic improvement in the level of pruritus. The owner assesses the itch score to be 3/10. The dog has one episode of vomiting during the first week of ciclosporin and has persistent soft stools. There is good hair regrowth on the ventral abdomen and ventral thorax. The axillae and groin have persistent hyperpigmentation and lichenification. Acetate strip cytology from the periocular areas, axillae and groin is unremarkable. The frequency of ciclosporin medication is reduced to alternate day dosing. The owners are shown the dog's normal gums and asked to check for gingival hyperplasia on an intermittent basis.

Eight weeks later there is a further improvement in the level of pruritus. The owner feels that the dog has a normal low level of itch (1/10) and is bright and active. The stools are occasionally soft, but otherwise well formed. The frequency of ciclosporin dosing is reduced to two non-consecutive days each week. The ventral hyperpigmentation has faded to a grey colour and the skin is only mildly thickened. There is a persistent pattern of mild surface corrugation in the axillae.

Eight weeks later the dog is bright and well, with only occasional licking of the front paws. There is mild erythema of the pad margins on a few of the digital pads on the front paws. There is only faint hyperpigmentation on the ventral abdomen and in the axillae, and the skin feels smooth.

Prognosis

The prognosis is good, but the dog is likely to need ongoing care, monitoring and medication.

Discussion

The dog in this case had two dietary trials to investigate a possible adverse food reaction. It is estimated that 10–25% of dogs with allergic skin disease have a food component to their hypersensitivity. It is very important to identify these individuals, as their skin disease may be resolved or improved without the need for unwarranted lifelong medication. A novel protein diet can be a cheaper and more readily available option than a hydrolysed diet, however, some commercial novel protein diets have been shown to be contaminated with animal protein, or proteins, that are not declared on the label. It is not known what dose of allergen is needed to trigger an adverse food reaction in the dog. Home cooking of novel proteins may avoid the cross contamination that may occur during manufacturing, but needs careful attention to hygiene, preparation and storage to avoid the same problem in the home kitchen. Many proteins are cross-reactive and it may be difficult to select appropriate ingredients for a food trial.

Allergic conjunctivitis and blepharitis are frequently seen aspects of atopic and atopic-like dermatitis in the dog. Blepharitis can partially occlude the punctae at the medial canthus, which normally provide a route for tear drainage down into the nose. Inflammation of the conjunctiva is associated with increased tear production. The combination of reduced tear drainage and increased tear production leads to overflow onto the skin. Persistent wetting and skin maceration can reduce the barrier function of the skin and the warm wet environment supports bacterial overgrowth.

High numbers of bacteria on the skin in the absence of neutrophils are likely to be a bacterial overgrowth rather than a superficial bacterial pyoderma. It is possible, but less likely, that they are contamination from an exogenous source. A bacterial overgrowth only involves the most superficial part of the epidermis and the skin surface, therefore topical treatment is a more logical and effective therapy in this situation than systemic antibiotics.

Bacterial overgrowth around the eyes can be treated with topical medication. It is important to avoid chlorhexidine-containing products as these can be damaging to the cornea. Suitable options include hypochlorous acid and povidone iodine solution. Hypochlorous acid has good antimicrobial activity but no residual action on the skin, making it more effective when applied several times each day. Povidone iodine solution can be used at a 1 : 50 dilution for intraocular lavage or a 1 : 10 dilution for cleansing the periocular skin. The 10% w/w cutaneous solution is used, not the detergent scrub formulation. Povidone iodine has a residual action and can be used once or twice daily. Owners should be warned that the product occasionally causes staining to pale coloured hair coats.

Ciclosporin causes vomiting in approximately one in four dogs and soft stools or diarrhoea in one in five dogs. If gastrointestinal signs occur they are usually mild and transient, as in this case.

Further reading

Horwath-Ungerboeck, C., Widmann, K., and Handl, S. (2017). Detection of DNA from undeclared animal species in commercial elimination diets for dogs using PCR. *Veterinary Dermatology* 28: 373–376.

Marsella, R. and De Benedetto, A. (2017). Atopic dermatitis in animals and people: an update and comparative review. *Veterinary Sciences* 4: 37–56.

Olivry, T. and Mueller, R. (2017). Critically appraised topic on adverse food reactions of companion animals (3): prevalence of cutaneous adverse food reactions in dogs and cats. *BMC Veterinary Research* 13: 51–54.

History

A 3 year-old female entire Large Munsterlander presents with a 1-month history of pruritus. The pruritus started suddenly at a moderate level and has increased to the current severe level. The dog spends a lot of time biting at the elbows and hocks, scratching the ears and head and dragging the ventrum along the ground. She also turns suddenly to bite at the abdomen. The owner is particularly concerned that the dog is restless and scratching during the night. The owner has a few red papules on both forearms. These very itchy lesions have appeared on the owner in the past few days. The other dog in the household is mildly pruritic and the owners are giving it chlorpheniramine twice daily. The five cats that share the household have no apparent pruritus or skin lesions. All of the animals receive occasional simultaneous topical fipronil for flea control. The skin lesions and the level of pruritus have been unchanged through treatment with a course of potentiated amoxicillin, topical ear medication and chlorhexidine-based shampoo.

Questions

1. Describe the abnormalities and pertinent normal features in Figures 16.1–16.4.
2. What differential diagnoses should be considered for this presentation?
3. What tests could you perform to make the diagnosis?

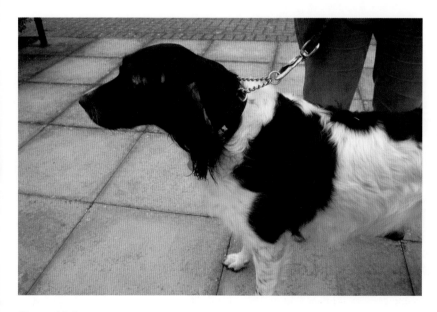

Figure 16.1

Small Animal Dermatology: What's Your Diagnosis? First Edition. Jane Coatesworth.
© 2019 John Wiley & Sons, Inc. Published 2019 by John Wiley & Sons, Inc.

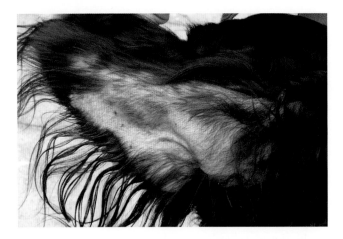

Figure 16.2

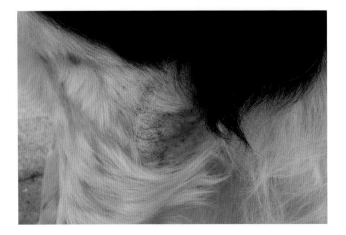

Figure 16.3

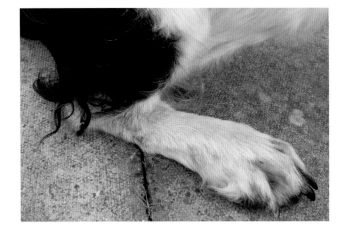

Figure 16.4

Answers

1. What the figures show

Figure 16.1 shows the left side of the dog. There are patches of hair loss and erythema caudal to the left eye, at the caudal aspect of the left ear and over the left elbow. The dog has a depressed demeanour.

Figure 16.2 shows the convex aspect of the left pinna. There is an extensive area of total and partial alopecia over the caudal two-thirds of the pinna, with a few erythematous papules, diffuse erythema and some excoriation.

Figure 16.3 shows a wide area of partial alopecia around the left lateral elbow. The skin is erythematous. The lichenification and hyperkeratosis over the pressure point of the elbow is a chronic change and pre-exists the recent skin problem.

Figure 16.4 shows the lateral aspect of the right hind limb. Moderate diffuse erythema is visible on the white haired distal limb. There is an area of barbered and broken hairs, erythematous papules and self-excoriation at the lateral hock. The interdigital skin is inflamed and alopecic.

2. Differential diagnoses

Given the appearance of the skin lesions the following conditions should be considered:

- Sarcoptic mange
- Ectopic *Otodectes* infestation. *Otodectes* mites can cause local skin irritation around the ears, and on the neck, caudal dorsum and tail. Mites are thought to transfer from the ears by direct contact when the animal is curled up, or is in direct contact with other infested animals. There is only a pruritic dermatosis if the individual animal has a hypersensitivity response to the mites on the skin.
- *Cheyletiella* infestation. The degree of pruritus associated with cheyletiellosis is very variable and can be severe. Cheyletiellosis typically has a truncal distribution and visible scaling, neither of which are present in this case.
- Allergic skin disease. The presence of pruritus affecting the face and feet in this young dog could be consistent with atopic dermatitis, but the involvement of the convex aspects of the pinnae and lateral elbows would not be typical. *Sarcoptes* mites have a number of common cross-reacting allergens with house dust mites, so it is important to make a clinical diagnosis of atopic dermatitis rather than one based on serological testing.

3. Appropriate diagnostic tests

Otoscopic examination and *cytology from a sample of ear wax* is unremarkable. *Skin scrapings* for evidence of *Sarcoptes* or *Cheyletiella*. A *Sarcoptes* infestation can be confirmed by finding mites, their eggs and/or their faecal pellets. Multiple superficial scrapings should be taken over a wide area, especially at the site of erythematous or crusted papules on thinly haired skin. The caudal pinna, when clinically affected, is a good place to start. Several *Sarcoptes* eggs are found, but no adult mites. No *Cheyletiella* mites or eggs are found.

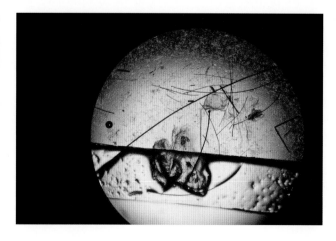

Figure 16.5 Shows a low power microscope image of material collected from a skin scraping. The sample is taken from of the caudal margin of the left pinna and mounted in liquid paraffin. The broad dark line running across the image is the edge of the glass coverslip. Three brown oval *Sarcoptes* eggs are clustered together just above the line and three more are distributed below the line.

Diagnosis

Sarcoptic mange.

Treatment

The affected dog and the in contact dog are given a spot-on formulation of selamectin, repeating the drug application after 4 weeks. Oclacitinib, at 0.5 mg kg^{-1} every 12 hours for 14 days, is dispensed for symptomatic relief. The degree of pruritus often increases shortly after miticidal treatment, probably due to the release of allergens from dead mites. Owner expectation needs to be managed around this time and concurrent antipruritic medication can be very helpful.

The owner is advised to seek medical attention for their own skin lesions. They are given a written report of their dog's skin condition in case it is helpful for their medical practitioner.

An acaricidal spray is dispensed for use in the house and car, as *Sarcoptes* mites can survive for a few days off the host and could be a potential source of infestation for other animals and people. Dog coats, grooming brushes and other potential fomites should also be cleaned and sprayed.

Prognosis

The prognosis is excellent for a full recovery if the dog is given appropriate treatment.

Discussion

A variety of drugs are available for the treatment of sarcoptic mange. This case was treated with topical selamectin in a spot-on formulation. Studies show that around 95% of dogs with *Sarcoptes* infestation have no detectable mites after a single application of selamectin, and 100% have no detectable mites after two applications separated by 1 month. A moxidectin/imidacloprid spot-on formulation is also effective at killing mites. Other treatment options include the isoxazolines afoxolaner, fluralaner, lotilaner and sarolaner. Afoxolaner, fluralaner and sarolaner have published studies showing efficacy against *Sarcoptes*, but only sarolaner is currently licensed in the United Kingdom for treatment of *Sarcoptes* acariasis. The scabies mite only burrows in the superficial layers of the epidermis so topical treatments can be effective, including amitraz or lime sulfur dips. Fipronil 0.25% w/v spray is useful for young infested puppies that are too small or too young to receive other products. It can be used from 2 days of age, taking care to avoid the eyes and to provide good ventilation until the product has dried on the coat.

The diagnosis in this case is made with a compatible history, typical clinical signs and the identification of *Sarcoptes* eggs on cytology. The total number of *Sarcoptes* mites affecting an individual dog is usually low, so it is important to recognise eggs and faecal pellets as well as the distinctive mites. The low number of *Sarcoptes* mites in an affected individual is in sharp contrast to the very high level of pruritus. Sarcoptic mange is typically a severely pruritic condition. The disparity between mite numbers and the degree of itch is due to the pruritus being partially the result of a hypersensitivity reaction to mite allergens and not just the result of the physical skin disruption caused by the burrowing mites. A small number of cases have very high mites numbers associated with extensive crusting and little pruritus. These animals should be checked for underlying causes of a compromised immune response.

Sarcoptes is potentially zoonotic and the pruritic papules that affect the owner in this case are likely to be caused by mites from the dog. Sarcoptic acariasis in dogs is caused by the host adapted strain *Sarcoptes scabiei* var. *canis*. These mites can burrow into the skin of in contact people, feed and lay eggs, but such infestations are only transient and self-limiting in healthy people. The human host adapted *S. scabiei* var. *hominis* can cause persistent infestations in people, but not in dogs. Cats are rarely affected by *S. scabiei* var. *canis*. The in-contact cats in this case are only monitored for possible clinical signs and not treated.

Further reading

Shanks, D.J., McTier, T.L., Behan, S. et al. (2000). The efficacy of selamectin in the treatment of naturally acquired infestations of *Sarcoptes scabiei* on dogs. *Veterinary Parasitology* 91: 269–281.

History

A 2 year-old female neutered domestic shorthaired cat presents with a 10 month history of excessive grooming and hair loss. The cat lives with a full litter sister that has no skin lesions or skin irritation. Both cats have been with the same owner since 7 weeks of age. They have an indoor/outdoor lifestyle and eat a commercial diet of open formula wet and dry food. The cats frequently supplement their diet by hunting for rodents and birds. They receive regular deworming and vaccination, and monthly flea control with selamectin spot-on. The house is sprayed regularly with an insecticidal spray. The owner sees the cat licking, biting and chewing at the hair coat and skin over much of the body, but especially at the ventral abdomen. The condition is unresponsive to three courses of antibiotics. The pruritic behaviour reduces significantly with long or short acting injectable glucocorticoids, but recurs as the medication wears off. Oral medication is not an option for this cat due to poor compliance.

Questions

1. Describe the abnormalities and pertinent normal features in Figures 17.1–17.4.
2. What differential diagnoses should be considered for this presentation?
3. What tests could you perform to make the diagnosis?

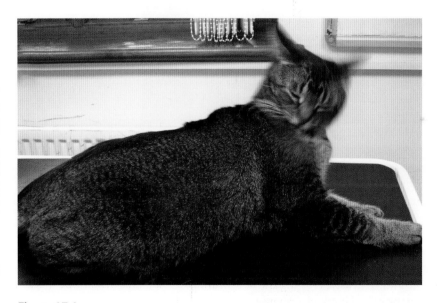

Figure 17.1

Small Animal Dermatology: What's Your Diagnosis? First Edition. Jane Coatesworth.
© 2019 John Wiley & Sons, Inc. Published 2019 by John Wiley & Sons, Inc.

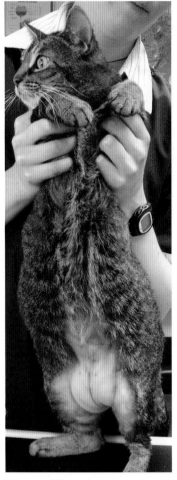

Figure 17.2

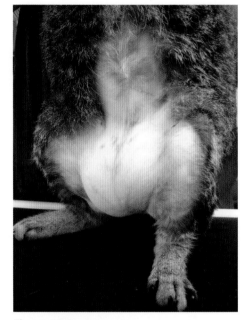

Figure 17.3

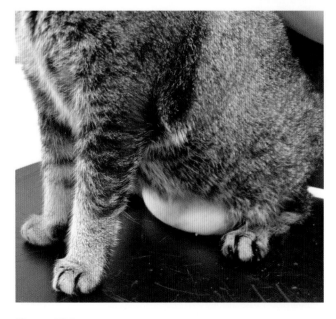

Figure 17.4

Answers

1. What the figures show

Figure 17.1 shows the cat during the consultation. The cat shows intermittent and very vigorous washing behaviour, directed at the neck, shoulders and forelimbs. There is a small patch of alopecia on the mid-lateral right forelimb. There are a few patches of short and broken guard hairs over the right lateral torso revealing the red/brown undercoat.

Figure 17.2 shows the ventral aspect of the cat. There is extensive and well demarcated alopecia of the ventral abdomen, groin and the proximal part of the medial hind limbs. The rest of the coat has a normal appearance.

Figure 17.3 shows a closer view of the alopecic ventral abdomen. There are focal areas of erythema and excoriation, especially around the nipples.

Figure 17.4 shows the left side of the cat. There are no obvious skin lesions, other than the prominent and alopecic fat pad lying between the hind limbs.

2. Differential diagnoses

Given the appearance of the skin lesions the following conditions should be considered:

- *Demodex gatoi*. These are short bodied *Demodex* mites that live in the superficial layers of the epidermis. They are particularly found on the ventral abdomen, flanks, inner thighs and forelimbs. Unlike the hair follicle based *Demodex cati*, *D. gatoi* can be both pruritic and contagious, and its presence is not associated with immunosuppression. The other cat in the household does not have any skin lesions, but this discrepancy has been seen between infected cats and may represent a variable degree of hypersensitivity to the mites.
- Flea bite hypersensitivity. This is a very common cause of pruritus in the cat.
- Cutaneous adverse food reaction (CAFR).
- Dermatophytosis has a highly pleomorphic clinical presentation and is a consideration in many feline cases.
- Atopic dermatitis.
- Generalised *Otodectes* infestation. This is unlikely as neither cat has no history of otitis, or of dark waxy material in the ears. *Otodectes* is generally contagious, but the degree of clinical signs varies between individuals and reflects a variable hypersensitivity response.
- Hyperthyroidism. This is unlikely as the cat is young, overweight and has a relaxed demeanour.
- Chronic cystitis causing local abdominal discomfort. Focal over-grooming of the ventral abdomen can be associated with underlying bladder inflammation. This cat shows generalised over-grooming behaviour, but urinalysis, which is a quick and economical test, is still justified here.

3. Appropriate diagnostic tests

General physical examination is unremarkable.

Wet paper test. Flea faeces have a high blood content. They leave a red/brown stain on damp white paper or cotton wool. No flea dirts are found in coat brushings from this cat.

Ear cytology and *otoscopic examination* are unremarkable.

Trichogram. Hair plucks from the margin of the alopecic areas show numerous fractured hair shafts, suggesting that hairs are being broken by trauma. This supports the owners history of over-grooming, and fits with the cat over-grooming during the consultation. There is a mixture of anagen and telogen bulbs, suggesting that the hair coat is capable of replacing itself.

Superficial skin scraping for *D. gatoi* and *faecal flotation* to recover ingested mites. Skin scrapings are also taken from the other cat in the household, but no *D. gatoi* are found. Adhesive tape strips can also be used to sample for this surface living mite.

Dermatophyte culture. The hair coat is examined with a Wood's lamp, but no foci of apple green fluorescence appear. It is helpful to pluck any bright fluorescent hairs that appear and use them for dermatophyte culture. In the absence of fluorescence, a sample for culture is obtained by brushing the cat with a sterile toothbrush. A sterile human scalp comb could also be used. The brush or comb picks up hairs and skin scale that can be transferred to the surface of dermatophyte culture medium. There is no dermatophyte growth in this case.

Urinalysis is unremarkable. The owners have never seen the cats urinate and the indoor litter tray is rarely used, so it is not possible to assess any behavioural signs of cystitis.

Food trial. Both cats are exclusively fed on a novel protein diet for an 8-week period. The trial is performed over the winter months, as the cats are more amenable to being kept indoors during this time. Symptomatic anti-pruritic medication is withdrawn towards the end of the food trial. The original diet is reintroduced at the end of the food trial. The owner reports an increase in the frequency of over-grooming towards the end of the food trial, probably related to the lack of symptomatic control. There is no change in the level of itch during the 2-week re-challenge period. This suggests that food allergens are not contributing to the pruritus.

Diagnosis

Atopic dermatitis. This diagnosis is made by the exclusion of other potential causes of pruritus, in this young and otherwise healthy cat.

Further diagnostic tests

IgE serology shows elevated IgE levels to storage mites (*Tyrophagus, Acarus*) and house dust mites (*Dermatophagoides farinae* and *Dermatophagoides pteronyssinus*).

Treatment

Regular flea control is recommended for both cats in the household. Topical selamectin is continued on a monthly basis, along with annual spraying of the indoor environment with an insecticidal spray. Most environmental flea sprays combine a rapid knockdown component with an insect growth inhibitor. As well as contributing to flea control, they cause a transient reduction in the house dust mite population. The cats are excluded from the bedrooms as these rooms generally have a high house dust mite population.

Allergen specific immunotherapy (ASIT) is given on a regular basis and the pruritus resolves after approximately 7 months of treatment. The cat continues to do well, over a 4-year follow up period, other than a return of pruritus when the immunotherapy is temporarily stopped due to household circumstances.

Prognosis

The prognosis is good for a good quality of life with ongoing treatment. Atopic dermatitis is a controllable but not a curable disease.

Discussion

ASIT is administered by injection, following a standard protocol where the dose volume increases and the time between the injections increases. Sublingual immunotherapy (SLIT) is also available but, as it is typically given twice daily this would not be an option for this uncooperative cat. The cat was given an alum precipitated immunotherapy vaccine, administered only once a month after completion of the loading phase. The clinical signs in this case resolve with immunotherapy alone, and recur on occasions when immunotherapy is temporarily stopped. Approximately 60% of cats will show a good response to ASIT. It is often helpful for owners to keep a diary of relevant clinical signs and degrees of pruritus. The diary can be periodically reviewed with the owner. Assessment of the overall response to treatment is usually assessed after at least a year of immunotherapy.

Dermatophytosis is a common cause of skin lesions in the cat. It presents with very variable lesions and levels of pruritus. The diagnosis is most robust when fluorescent hairs are found around the lesions, and a compatible dermatophyte grows on culture. However, only a proportion of *Microsporum canis* strains fluoresce under a Wood's lamp. Collecting hair and skin scale with a toothbrush or human scalp comb samples from a wide area. Some cats are transient asymptomatic carriers of dermatophytes. False positives can occur where the presence of dermatophyte contamination is unrelated to the skin lesions. A negative result, as in this case, is useful to rule out dermatophytosis.

The median prevalence of CAFR in cats with pruritus is thought to be between 15 and 20%. These substantial figures justify the effort and inconvenience of performing a food trial. In this case both cats in the household were fed the same novel protein diet, and were kept indoors to prevent supplementary food consumption including hunting. A food trial lasting 8 weeks will give complete remission of clinical signs in more than 90% of cats with CAFR.

Oral ciclosporin is widely available and licensed for use in feline chronic allergic dermatitis. The drug is available as a liquid formulation, but any form of oral medication is not an option for this cat. A small pilot study has looked at the use of injectable ciclosporin in 11 allergic cats. Cats were given 2.5 or 5 mg kg^{-1} of a 50 mg ml^{-1} injectable ciclosporin solution, daily or every other day, by subcutaneous injection. Five cats were withdrawn from the study at the request of the owner. Two had issues at the injection site reported by the owner, two had owners that were not comfortable continuing to give injections and one had behavioural changes and a lack of response to therapy reported by the owner. Six cats finished the 2-month study and they all showed a good clinical response.

Further reading

Olivry, T., Mueller, R.S., and Prélaud, P. (2015). Critically appraised topic on adverse food reactions of companion animals (1): duration of elimination diets. *BMC Veterinary Research* 11: 225–227.

Koch, S., Torres, S.M.F., Diaz, S. et al. (2018). Subcutaneous administration of ciclosporin in 11 allergic cats – a pilot open-label uncontrolled clinical trial. *Veterinary Dermatology* 29: 107–111.

Ravens, P.A. (2014). Feline atopic dermatitis: a retrospective study of 45 cases (2001–2012). *Veterinary Dermatology* 25: 95–102.

History

A 5 year-old female entire Border Collie cross presents with a history of swelling on the dorsal muzzle. The owner sees the dog rubbing at the muzzle and noticed 'a few small red bumps' 36 hours earlier. The extent and severity of the lesions has progressed rapidly since then. The dog is inappetent and a little lethargic. There is no previous history of skin disease.

Questions

1. Describe the abnormalities and pertinent normal features in Figures 18.1–18.3.
2. What differential diagnoses should be considered for this presentation?
3. What tests could you perform to make the diagnosis?

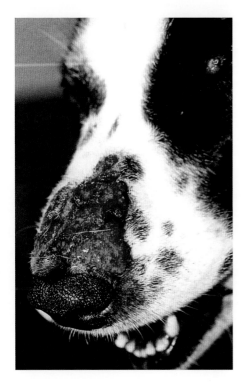

Figure 18.1

Small Animal Dermatology: What's Your Diagnosis? First Edition. Jane Coatesworth.
© 2019 John Wiley & Sons, Inc. Published 2019 by John Wiley & Sons, Inc.

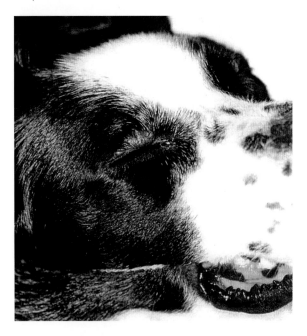

Figure 18.2

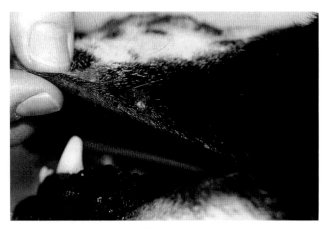

Figure 18.3

Answers

1. What the figures show

Figure 18.1 shows the dog's face. There is a well circumscribed, haemorrhagic, ulcerated, exudative and alopecic plaque on the rostro-dorsal muzzle. The plaque is adjacent to, but not involving, the nasal planum and a thin strip of normal haired skin is maintained between the two. There are several coalescing erythematous papules on the middle of the left upper eyelid and adjacent to the nasal planum below the left nostril.

Figure 18.2 shows the dog's face. There are oedematous and erythematous coalescing papules along 80% of the length of the right upper eyelid.

Figure 18.3 shows the left upper lip. There is an erythematous papule, approximately 6 mm in diameter, on the haired lip margin with a bead of overlying haemorrhagic exudate.

2. **Differential diagnoses**

Given the appearance of the skin lesions the following conditions should be considered:

- Eosinophilic folliculitis and furunculosis.
- Bacterial folliculitis and furunculosis of the dorsal muzzle is a condition of longer-nosed dogs. The coalescing papules, pustules, nodules and discharging sinuses are often pruritic. The condition may be initiated by trauma to the area, and perpetuated by the trauma of rubbing to assuage the irritation.
- Sterile granuloma/pyogranuloma syndrome. This uncommon condition can present with papules and plaques which subsequently ulcerate. The distribution of lesions typically includes the face, including the muzzle and periocular area. A granuloma is characterised by macrophages on cytology and histopathology, and a pyogranuloma by macrophages and neutrophils. No micro-organisms are expected in the sterile form.
- Drug eruption.
- Dermatophytosis forming a kerion. A kerion is usually a solitary lesion, but multiple lesions are occasionally reported. The classic kerion is circular and domed, alopecic, erythematous and well demarcated. Beads of serous or haemorrhagic fluid may form on the surface. There is rarely any associated pain or pruritus and the lesions usually resolve spontaneously.
- Contact irritant or contact allergic dermatitis. Contact reactions generally occur in thinly haired areas with an inadequate protective hair coat. There are erythematous papules or macules, and a significant degree of irritation.
- Pemphigus foliaceus.
- Pemphigus erythematosus.

3. **Appropriate diagnostic tests**

General physical examination is unremarkable. In addition to the lesions shown in the figures, smaller coalescing erythematous papules are present on the margin of the left pinna and adjacent to the nasal planum below the left nostril. The dog resents close examination of the lesions and the affected skin appears to be painful.

Cytology. Impression smears from the wet surface of the lesions show numerous eosinophils, a few neutrophils and no bacteria.

Skin biopsies are taken from the edge and the centre of the dorsal muzzle lesion and from the lip lesion. Two of the punch biopsies are taken without clipping and cleaning and are submitted in formalin for histopathology. The histopathology shows extensive ulceration of the epidermis. There is a dense infiltrate of inflammatory cells dominated by eosinophils throughout the depth of the dermis. Large numbers of aggregated eosinophils are present within intact hair follicles and at the site of ruptured follicles. No fungal elements or bacteria are seen on special stains. These findings support a diagnosis of eosinophilic folliculitis and furunculosis.

The other biopsy sample is taken with a sterile technique, after clipping and cleaning the area, and submitted for bacterial culture and sensitivity. There is no bacterial growth from the tissue sample.

Diagnosis

Eosinophilic folliculitis and furunculosis.

Treatment

Oral prednisolone is started after skin biopsy, at $1\,mg\,kg^{-1}$ once daily. This decision is based on the clinical likelihood of eosinophilic disease and the need to provide some symptomatic relief for this painful and pruritic condition.

Ten days later the biopsy sites have healed well and the sutures are removed. The eyelid, lip and pinnal lesions have resolved. The muzzle lesion is less swollen and less erythematous. The oral prednisolone is reduced to $1\,mg\,kg^{-1}$ on alternate days for 10 days, and then to $0.5\,mg\,kg^{-1}$ on alternate days.

Two weeks later some hair is re-growing on the dorsal muzzle and the active lesions have resolved. Prednisolone is discontinued.

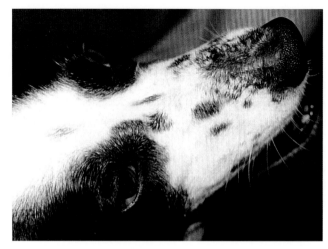

Figure 18.4 Shows scarring alopecia and hyperpigmentation on the rostro-dorsal muzzle 2 months after initial presentation.

Prognosis

There is an excellent prognosis for full recovery. The dog has a stable area of scarring alopecia 14 months after the initial onset. The condition may recur if the dog is exposed again to a similar allergenic trigger, however, this is uncommon and may reflect learning and behavioural changes in previously affected dogs.

Discussion

Eosinophilic folliculitis and furunculosis may be a peracute hypersensitivity response to arthropod bites or stings, and similar to mosquito bite hypersensitivity in the cat. This case occurred in July, when arthropods are numerous and active. The condition responded promptly to glucocorticoids. However, no insect or spider encounters were seen by the owner and no similar reactions were seen for the 5 years before, or during the year since this occasion. The arthropod bite or sting theory is supported by the distribution of lesions at the thinly haired areas of the head, and by documented cases occurring after witnessed interactions with bees, ants, spiders or wasps. Lesions on the trunk and distal limbs have also been reported.

The rapid progression of the disease can be alarming for owners, especially when there is no obvious inciting cause. The intensely erythematous papules, nodules and plaques quickly ulcerate and develop overlying areas of haemorrhagic crust. This dog has a moderate degree of pruritus and the affected areas appear to be painful on handling. The pruritus associated with this condition can vary from absent to severe. The majority of cases respond briskly to corticosteroid administration.

Further reading

Curtis, C., Bond, R., Blunden, A.S. et al. (1995). Canine eosinophilic folliculitis and furunculosis in three cases. *Journal of Small Animal Practice* 36: 119–123.

Mason, K. and Evans, A. (1991). Mosquito bite caused eosinophilic dermatitis in the cat. *Journal of the American Veterinary Medical Association* 198: 2086–2088.

History

A 7 year-old male neutered Newfoundland presents with a 1-year history of a pruritic and malodorous area on the ventral neck. The lesion started with small moist pink sores, which coalesced to form a large alopecic area. The extent of the affected area has fluctuated over the past 12 months but has never resolved. Skin swabs, taken for bacterial culture and sensitivity, have returned heavy growths of both *Proteus* spp. and *Pseudomonas aeruginosa* on two different occasions. The dog has received courses of oral potentiated amoxicillin, cephalexin, metronidazole and marbofloxacin, with little effect. The owner sees the dog regularly abrading the ventral neck by rubbing back and forth along furniture of a suitable height. The dog frequently licks and scratches at the affected skin, but has no history of generalised skin disease.

Questions

1. Describe the abnormalities and pertinent normal features in Figures 19.1 and 19.2.
2. What differential diagnoses should be considered for this presentation?
3. What tests could you perform to make the diagnosis?

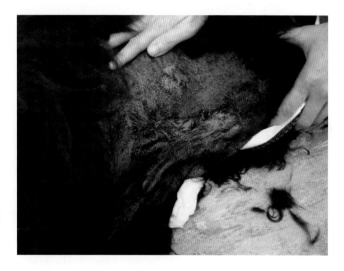

Figure 19.1

Small Animal Dermatology: What's Your Diagnosis? First Edition. Jane Coatesworth.
© 2019 John Wiley & Sons, Inc. Published 2019 by John Wiley & Sons, Inc.

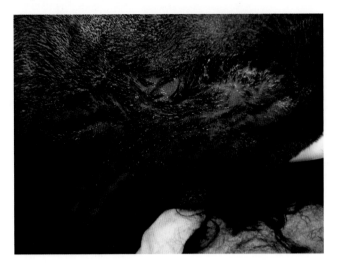

Figure 19.2

Answers

1. **What the figures show**

   Figure 19.1 shows the ventral neck area. The dog is sedated and in left lateral recumbency with the nose to the right of the photograph. The affected area is only visible when the neck folds are stretched apart laterally. The overlying wet, matted and adherent hair has been clipped away. A wide border of normal skin has also been clipped. The adherent gelatinous material on the skin surface and the surrounding dried crust have been gently and thoroughly washed away.

   Figure 19.2 shows a closer view of the ventral neck. There is an extensive area of eroded, swollen, hypotrichotic, erythematous and exudative skin within the recessed part of a deep ventral neck fold.

2. **Differential diagnoses**

   Given the appearance of the skin lesions the following conditions should be considered:

   - Pyotraumatic dermatitis. This condition is also known as a 'hot spot' or acute moist dermatitis. Bacteria are only present on the skin surface and in the first few layers of the epidermis. The lesion is well demarcated from the surrounding normal skin.
   - Pyotraumatic folliculitis and furunculosis. This presents as a palpably thicker lesion with bacteria invading the hair follicles and bacteria in the dermis after rupture of infected hair follicles. The lesions may be ill-defined, with surrounding erythematous papules and/or pustules.
   - Intertrigo is an inflammatory condition caused by friction and abrasion between two skin surfaces. It is often complicated by secondary bacterial and/or yeast overgrowth. Although the affected area in this case is enclosed by folds of skin on the ventral neck, the folds do not rub against each other but hang in parallel.
   - Hypothyroidism was considered in this middle-aged dog with a chronic non-healing skin lesion.

3. **Appropriate diagnostic tests**

   Physical examination reveals a 4/6 systolic murmur, which is audible on both sides of the thorax and difficult to localise. The dog is uncooperative and mildly aggressive when attempts are made to examine the ventral neck. He is sedated with 0.4 mg kg^{-1} butorphanol, by intravenous injection, to allow examination of the area.

   Cytology shows very high numbers of rod-shaped bacteria. Touching a clean glass slide onto the wet lesion produces helpful impression smears for Diff Quik staining. High bacterial numbers, in the absence of neutrophils, are suggestive of a bacterial overgrowth on the skin surface.

Total T4 and *thyroid stimulating hormone (TSH) assays* were within the normal range, excluding a diagnosis of hypothyroidism.

Diagnosis

Pyotraumatic dermatitis of the ventral neck.

Treatment

The initial treatment of the neck lesion is carried out while the dog is sedated. The residual hair coat is clipped short over the affected skin and to a 25 cm margin all around the lesion. Any hair that would trail onto the affected skin when the dog was in a normal position is also clipped short. The affected skin and the adjacent clipped normal skin are thoroughly washed with 2% chlorhexidine in a detergent scrub formulation. The skin is rinsed with water and blotted dry with absorbent paper. A solution of TrizEDTA is applied to the affected skin, left for 2 min and blotted dry. The area is covered in a thin layer of 1% w/w silver sulfadiazine cream. The owners are asked to wash the clipped area once daily, but to use a shampoo formulation of 2% chlorhexidine. TrizEDTA and silver sulfadiazine should be applied twice daily while there is a lot of exudate, then once daily when the area becomes drier. Meloxicam, at 0.1 mg kg^{-1} once daily by mouth, is dispensed for analgesia.

The owners are asked to only feed the dog twice daily and to stop giving treats in between meals. This change is an attempt to reduce the daily volume of salivation. The dog is excluded from the dining room when the owners are eating, as he tends to salivate more at these times.

The water bowls are emptied, cleaned and refilled on a regular basis, rather than being continuously topped up, to reduce their level of contamination with *Pseudomonas* bacteria.

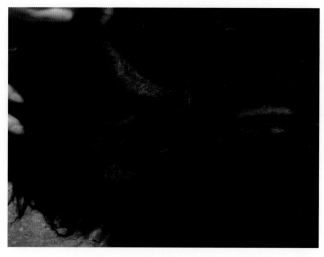

Figure 19.3 Shows the ventral neck with the neck fold held open after 4 weeks of treatment. The dog is in right lateral recumbency with the nose to the left. The dog is not sedated and does not react to handling of the area. There is limited visible hair regrowth as the owner has been able to re-clip the affected area, with good cooperation from the dog. The skin has a normal pink/grey colour.

The owners report that the dog is more comfortable within 1 day of starting treatment. This rapid relief may be associated with the meloxicam and the removal of long hair that was contacting the sensitive lesion. The skin is noticeably drier and less red after 1 week of treatment. The owners feel that the lesion resolved after 3 weeks and they discontinued the treatment. The owners will keep the hair coat clipped short on the ventral neck and monitor the area regularly so that any recurrence can be treated at an early stage.

Prognosis

The prognosis is good, but the condition can recur if there is not adequate control of the predisposing factors.

Discussion

Pyotraumatic dermatitis is often started by self-trauma, in response to a pruritic focus. It has an acute onset and can progress rapidly. The location can be suggestive of the initial cause, for example adjacent to inflamed ears or impacted anal sacs. Flea infestation, allergic dermatitis, local joint pain or soft tissue injury are common trigger factors. Pyotraumatic dermatitis commonly begins, as in this case, during a period of hot weather. Large breed dogs with a dense secondary coat, such as this Newfoundland, are predisposed. The Golden Retriever, German Shepherd dog and Saint Bernard are commonly affected, but any breed can be affected.

Pseudomonas aeruginosa bacteria are widespread in the environment and are opportunistic colonisers of moist skin. They are particularly successful in persistently warm and wet skin environments that lead to maceration. Factors in this case that support the growth of *Pseudomonas* are likely to include the dense matted hair coat, the initial period of warm weather, the deep skin folds, the skin inflammation and exudation and the persistent drooling that is common in the breed. Wet lip folds can harbour significant populations of *Pseudomonas* in dogs with unhelpful lip conformation. Pyotraumatic dermatitis, associated with *Pseudomonas* overgrowth, can be seen on the dewlap of rabbits with dental problems and associated excessive drooling.

Pseudomonas readily covers the skin with a layer of biofilm. Biofilm is a highly organised cooperative colony of bacteria that is surrounded by a protective matrix layer largely consisting of polysaccharides. The protective matrix gives enhanced resistance to physical disruption, antiseptics and antibiotics. A proportion of the bacteria within a biofilm have very slow rates of cell division, adding to the colony's resistance to antibiotics. Physical cleansing and disruption of the biofilm are important aspects of successful treatment, hence the use of thorough physical washing and a detergent formulation of chlorhexidine for the first cleaning in this case, and the regular use of TrizEDTA. Staphylococcal overgrowth is generally much more common in pyotraumatic dermatitis in the dog than overgrowth by *Pseudomonas* spp. Cytology is a fast and inexpensive method to check whether cocci or rods are present.

Clipping the overlying and surrounding hair coat allows better visualisation and assessment of the lesion. Clipping also removes contaminated hair, and improves local access and ease of skin cleaning. Pyotraumatic dermatitis usually responds well to appropriate topical treatment and, unlike pyotraumatic folliculitis and furunculosis, systemic antibiotics are not indicated. This case received several courses of systemic antibiotics with no apparent effect. *Pseudomonas aeruginosa* has an impressive array of antibiotic resistance mechanisms. The bacterial outer wall has low permeability to antibiotics and any antibiotic that gets into the cell is readily removed by efflux pumps. The bacteria can modify the sites of antibiotic action, making them unrecognisable, and can produce enzymes that neutralise antibiotics in their immediate surroundings.

This dog has an extensive lesion and is showing signs of significant pruritus and pain. A non-steroidal anti-inflammatory drug is used to improve the dog's welfare, to reduce the inflammation in the lesion and to allow the owners to safely and effectively treat the affected area at home. Pain, pruritus and inflammation can be reduced using topical corticosteroids, such as hydrocortisone aceponate spray. A gel containing betamethasone and fusidic acid can be helpful for cases of pyotraumatic dermatitis with staphylococcal involvement.

Cases of pyotraumatic dermatitis usually respond well to topical therapy in 1 or 2 weeks. In this very chronic case there was resolution after 3 weeks of topical therapy. The initial trigger is unknown in this case, which makes recurrence an unquantifiable risk. Keeping the hair coat short, monitoring the area and reducing the degree of skin wetting are all likely to be helpful in the long term.

Further reading

Holm, B.R., Rest, J.R., and Seewald, W. (2004). A prospective study of the clinical findings, treatment and histopathology of 44 cases of pyotraumatic dermatitis. *Veterinary Dermatology* 15: 369–376.

Cobb, M.A., Edwards, H.J., Jagger, T.D. et al. (2005). Topical fusidic acid/betamethasone-containing gel compared to systemic therapy in the treatment of canine acute moist dermatitis. *The Veterinary Journal* 169: 276–280.

Schroeder, H., Swan, G.E., Berry, W.L., and Pearson, J. (1996). Efficacy of a topical antimicrobial-anti-inflammatory combination in the treatment of pyotraumatic dermatitis in dogs. *Veterinary Dermatology* 7: 163–170.

Viking Höglund, O. and Frendin, J. (2002). Analgesic effect of meloxicam in canine acute dermatitis – a pilot study. *Acta Veterinaria Scandinavica* 43: 247–252.

History

A 2 year-old female neutered German Shepherd dog is presented with a 2-month history of pruritus. Neither of the owners or the second dog in the household have any history of skin problems. The dog has lived with the owners since 12 weeks of age and has not travelled overseas. Pruritus started with rubbing of the face and head shaking and progressed to generalised scratching and rubbing. The owners also see and hear regular episodes of chewing all four feet, licking of the abdomen and gnawing at the perineum.

Questions

1. Describe the abnormalities and pertinent normal features in Figures 20.1–20.4.
2. What differential diagnoses should be considered for this presentation?
3. What tests could you perform to make the diagnosis?

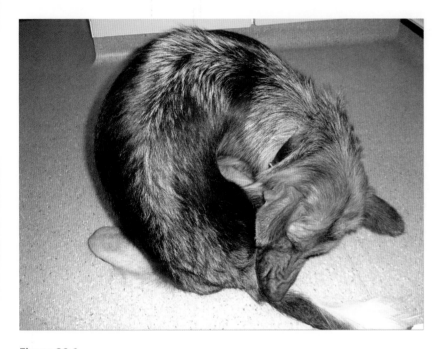

Figure 20.1

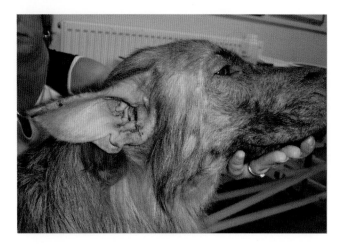

Figure 20.2

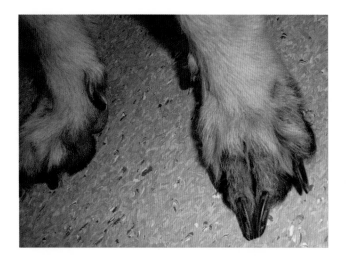

Figure 20.3

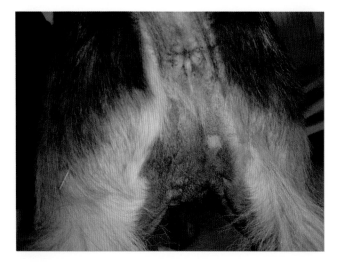

Figure 20.4

Answers

1. What the figures show

Figure 20.1 shows the dog using the incisor teeth to gnaw at the tail base. This, and other types of pruritic behaviour, are persistently displayed during the initial consultation. There is erythema and alopecia of the muzzle, the medial left stifle and the outer aspect of the right pinna.

Figure 20.2 shows erythema and partial alopecia of the convex aspect of the right pinna, periocular skin and face. Both ears have a mild waxy discharge. Areas of recent self-excoriation can be seen on the pinnal margin and at the commissures of the lips. There is hyperpigmentation at the base of the ear and around the eye.

Figure 20.3 shows marked erythema and alopecia of the digits and the pad margins of both front feet. There is hyperpigmentation at and adjacent to the nailbeds. Similar changes are seen on the hind feet.

Figure 20.4 shows alopecia, hyperpigmentation and lichenification of the perineum and ventral tail base. There are focal patches of erythema and excoriation.

2. Differential diagnoses

Given the appearance of the skin lesions, the following conditions should be considered:

- Atopic dermatitis
- Atopic-like dermatitis
- Fleabite hypersensitivity
- Cutaneous adverse food reaction
- Sarcoptic mange
- Demodectic mange with secondary bacterial infection
- Superficial bacterial pyoderma
- *Malassezia* otitis externa
- Bacterial otitis externa

3. Appropriate diagnostic tests

General *physical examination* shows enlargement of the popliteal and pre-scapular lymph nodes. Peripheral lymphadenopathy is a variable feature of generalised inflammatory skin disease and is most commonly associated with generalised demodicosis.

Dermatological examination, further to the lesions shown in the photographs, reveals alopecia of the ventral abdomen, medial hind limbs and axillae. The palmar and plantar interdigital spaces are alopecic and severely erythematous. The skin of the medial thighs is lichenified and hyperpigmented. The pinnal margins are crusted in places. Erythematous papules, crusted papules and epithelial collarettes are seen on the ventral abdomen.

Cytology from both ears showed high numbers of *Malassezia*, an occasional coccus and no inflammatory cells.

A touch impression, from beneath the crust of a crusted papule, showed degenerate neutrophils with both intracytoplasmic and free cocci. The presence of intracytoplasmic bacteria confirms that a bacterial infection is present.

Acetate tape impressions from the interdigital spaces are unremarkable.

Deep and *superficial skin scrapings* from lesional skin, including the crusted pinnal margins, showed no *Sarcoptes* or *Demodex* mites. *Demodex* mites are relatively easy to see in deep skin scrapes, other than in the SharPei where excess dermal mucin can make diagnostic scraping impossible. *Sarcoptes* mites can be much more challenging to find than *Demodex* mites and serology is a useful additional test when the clinical suspicion is high.

A *serology* sample for *Sarcoptes* IgG returns results within the normal range. This result is helpful as we are suspicious of atopic dermatitis in this case. *Sarcoptes* can cross react with house dust mite serology and intradermal testing, so a negative *Sarcoptes* serology allows us to interpret positive house dust mite results with more confidence.

A strict *elimination diet* was started, using a commercial dry complete diet containing fish and potato. The dog had not been previously fed a diet containing fish or potato. The owner declined the option of preparing a home-cooked diet. Although a home-cooked diet is likely to contain fewer allergens than a commercial diet, many owners are unable or unwilling to follow this option.

Working diagnosis

Atopic (or atopic-like) dermatitis and/or cutaneous adverse food reaction, with concurrent superficial bacterial pyoderma and bilateral *Malassezia* otitis externa.

Treatment

Clindamycin was dispensed at $11\,mg\,kg^{-1}$ once daily for a 3-week course. Clindamycin is a suitable first line antibiotic choice for superficial bacterial pyoderma. It has good activity against staphylococci in our geographical area, although local antibiotic resistance patterns can vary. The once-daily dosing is helpful for owner compliance. The owners are asked to bath the dog twice each week in a chlorhexidine based shampoo, until the next examination, and to use a moderately ceruminolytic ear cleaner once daily for 2 weeks.

Chlorpheniramine is dispensed at $0.25\,mg\,kg^{-1}$ every 12 hours for a 2-week course. Antihistamines have a low overall efficacy as antipruritic drugs, but can be helpful in individual cases and can have a steroid sparing effect. Chlorpheniramine is a first generation antihistamine and may cause sedation. Oclacitinib or glucocorticoids could be more reliable alternatives here, as short acting antipruritic agents, to give symptomatic relief.

Telephone discussion 2 weeks later confirms that the dog is cooperating with the tablets, the bathing and the diet and is free of spots on the abdomen.

Further testing and outcome

Six weeks later the owner reports an approximately 25% reduction in pruritus. There was no deterioration in pruritus when the chlorpheniramine was stopped after 2 weeks, suggesting minimal impact from this drug. Examination shows alopecia and moderate erythema of the palmar and plantar interdigital spaces, the metacarpal and metatarsal areas, the dorsal paws, concave pinnae, ventral abdomen and groin. There is partial hair regrowth at the other previously affected sites. The superficial bacterial pyoderma has not recurred and cytology from both ears is unremarkable.

An *intradermal test* is performed under medetomidine sedation and shows an immediate positive reaction only to the histamine positive control. A blood sample is taken for immunoglobulin E (IgE) serology and gives no positive results. Antihistamines and glucocorticoids should be discontinued at least 2 weeks before intradermal testing as they can suppress positive reactions.

The owner is asked to feed the elimination diet for a further 2 weeks, to then re-challenge with all aspects of the original diet and to monitor the level of pruritus for the subsequent 2 weeks. Twice weekly bathing is continued. Telephone discussion 4 weeks later reveals no further improvement on completion of the elimination diet and no change in pruritus during the 2 weeks back on the regular diet. This suggests that food intolerance is not part of the dog's hypersensitivity condition.

Oral prednisolone is dispensed at $0.5\,mg\,kg^{-1}$ once daily for 10 days, then reducing to $0.5\,mg\,kg^{-1}$ every other day. The chlorhexidine bathing is reduced to once weekly.

A further 6 weeks later the owner reports a comfortable dog with intermittent nibbling at all four feet. Examination shows good hair regrowth at all of the previously alopecic areas.

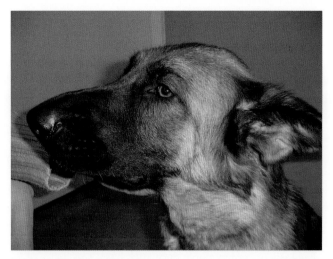

Figure 20.5 Shows the dog after controlling secondary infections and after 6 weeks of treatment with oral prednisolone. There is good hair regrowth over the head and pinna. There is only a small remaining area of alopecia at the base of the left ear.

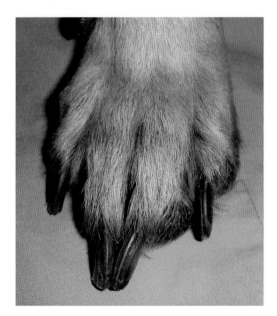

Figure 20.6 Shows the left front foot after 6 weeks of treatment with oral prednisolone. There is hair regrowth at the previously alopecic areas. The underlying skin has persistent hyperpigmentation but is no longer erythematous. Long nails are a common feature of inflammatory pododermatitis, as there is increased blood supply to the nail beds.

Fourteen months later the dog is maintained on low dose alternate day prednisolone and whole body bathing every 2 weeks. Prednisolone is generally well tolerated at or below a dose of 0.5 mg kg^{-1} every other day. The medication is usually given to dogs in the morning with food. A steroid sparing effect has been demonstrated for essential fatty acid supplementation with Viacutan (Boeringer) and may occur with other similar products. Dogs on long term steroid treatment have an increased risk of occult urinary tract infections and need intermittent urinalysis to identify these. Dogs on low dose alternate day prednisolone can have their routine annual vaccinations without a break of medication.

Final diagnosis

Atopic-like dermatitis.

Prognosis

There is a variable prognosis, depending on the long term response to treatment.

Discussion

Atopic (and atopic-like) dermatitis is a clinical diagnosis. Diagnosis is not always easy as the condition can present with a variety of clinical signs. The clinical signs can all be shared by other diseases, requiring a careful process of exclusion to produce the diagnosis. The exclusion of diseases with similar signs is combined with the recognition of characteristic clinical features. A number of diagnostic criteria have been proposed over the years to aid in the diagnosis of canine atopic dermatitis and for use in clinical trials. The most recent, and perhaps most helpful set of diagnostic criteria were published in 2010 by Favrot et al. Using these criteria, a diagnosis of canine atopic dermatitis has a specificity of 79%, and a sensitivity of 85% if five of the eight criteria are met. Although diagnostic criteria can be helpful for critical assessment of clinical signs in our patients, we need to remember that one in five dogs that satisfy 5/8 Favrot criteria will *not* have atopic dermatitis.

Favrot diagnostic criteria for canine atopic dermatitis

At least five of the eight criteria are required. The dog in this case has seven of the eight criteria.

- Onset of clinical signs under 3 years of age
- Dog living mostly indoors
- Corticosteroid responsive pruritus
- Chronic or recurrent yeast infections
- Affected front feet
- Affected ear pinnae
- Non-affected ear margins
- Non-affected dorso-lumbar area

Atopic-like dermatitis has been defined as an inflammatory and pruritic skin disease with clinical features identical to those seen in canine atopic dermatitis. In atopic-like dermatitis an IgE response to environmental or other allergens cannot be documented. No allergens were identified in this case, either on serology or intradermal testing. Some people with atopic dermatitis have no response to skin tests and no excess IgE production. So-called 'intrinsic' atopy in people may have alternative immunological pathways and a similar situation may be occurring in a proportion of atopic dogs. Management with allergen specific immunotherapy and allergen avoidance is not an option for dogs with atopic-like dermatitis.

The food trial in this case was conducted for 8 weeks. In a trial of 51 dogs, Rosser showed that 94% of food intolerant dogs had a positive response to food trial after 8 weeks, while only 74% responded after 6 weeks. A home-cooked or hydrolysate diet may have given superior results in this case, but the owner declined the first and the dog refused the second. Fish and potato was chosen as a novel protein and carbohydrate source based on the previous dietary history.

Secondary microbial infection is a common feature of atopic dermatitis. In this case, the degree of pruritus improved by 25% after resolution of the *Malassezia* otitis and the bacterial superficial pyoderma. The dog was still, however, significantly above its pruritic threshold. The reduction in pruritus was judged not to be related to the change of diet, as there was no subsequent increase in pruritus on food re-challenge. A diagnosis of food intolerance needs to have all three diagnostic components present; namely, improvement on a food trial, relapse on food challenge and improvement again on a food trial.

The dog's pruritus is responsive to a low dose of corticosteroids, in combination with regular antimicrobial bathing. There is a good response to treatment after 10 days, so the dose is reduced to a sustainable alternate day dose to maintain the effect. Oral prednisolone is effective approximately four hours after ingestion making it suitable for the initial control of skin inflammation and for the treatment of acute flares, as well as for low dose alternate day maintenance therapy.

There is increasing evidence that atopic dogs have poor skin barrier function in comparison to non-atopic individuals. Regular bathing may be helpful in reducing the cutaneous load of microbes, inflammatory mediators and allergens. Secondary cutaneous bacterial and yeast infections are common flare factors in canine atopic dermatitis and are best prevented rather than treated reactively on a frequent basis.

Further reading

Halliwell, R. (2006). Revised nomenclature for veterinary allergy. *Veterinary Immunology and Immunopathology* 114: 207–208.

Favrot, C., Steffan, J., Seewald, W., and Picco, F. (2010). A prospective study on the clinical features of chronic canine atopic dermatitis and its diagnosis. *Veterinary Dermatology* 21: 23–31.

Olivry, T. and Hill, P.B. (2001). American College of Veterinary Dermatology Taskforce on canine atopic dermatitis: is the epidermal lipid barrier defective? *Veterinary Immunology and Immunopathology* 81: 215–218.

Rosser, E.J. (1993). Diagnosis of food allergy in dogs. *Journal of the American Veterinary Medical Association* 203: 259–262.

Torres, S., Diaz, S.F., Nogueira, S.A. et al. (2005). Frequency of urinary tract infection among dogs with pruritic disorders receiving long term glucocorticoid treatment. *Journal of the American Veterinary Medical Association* 227: 239–243.

Pustules, Crust and Scale

A *pustule* is a small discrete pocket of pus with a rounded surface contour. Pustules form within the layers of the epidermis or in hair follicles. Pus contains a high proportion of white blood cells, either neutrophils and/or eosinophils, which confer the typical creamy yellow colour. Pustules that form in hair follicles are likely to be associated with a bacterial folliculitis, or more rarely caused by dermatophytosis. The commonest type of pustule contains neutrophils and is associated with bacterial skin disease. Neutrophilic pustules can also contain no bacteria, such as in the large sterile non-follicular pustules associated with pemphigus foliaceus or leishmaniosis.

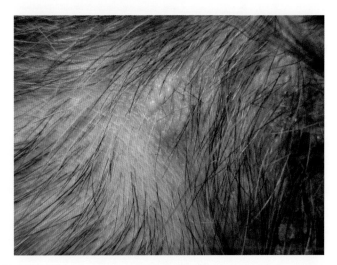

Figure D.1 Shows a thinly haired area caudal to the right elbow of a young terrier cross. There are three non-follicular pustules in a line and a cluster of smaller pustules below them. There are crusts and erosions to the right of the photograph where pustules have recently ruptured. This dog has pemphigus foliaceus, and the pustules are neutrophilic and sterile.

Pustules that contain eosinophils are found in the rare pruritic condition sterile eosinophilic pustulosis and occasionally in dogs with flea bite hypersensitivity. Eosinophils may be seen, along with the neutrophils, in cytology samples from the pustules of pemphigus foliaceus.

Large pustules that span numerous hair follicles are most commonly seen in pemphigus foliaceus, impetigo in puppies and with immunosuppressive diseases such as hyperadrenocorticism. Pustules are soft and have a domed roof comprising only a thin layer of cells. They are quick to rupture and dehydrate, and are relatively short lived lesions. Feline skin is even thinner than canine skin and the pustular stage of a disease is rarely observed in the cat.

Small Animal Dermatology: What's Your Diagnosis? First Edition. Jane Coatesworth.
© 2019 John Wiley & Sons, Inc. Published 2019 by John Wiley & Sons, Inc.

Scale is a visible flake of dead exfoliated skin cells. Skin cells are normally and constantly shed from the skin surface in small imperceptible units, so the presence of visible scale reflects a change in the normal pattern of skin turnover.

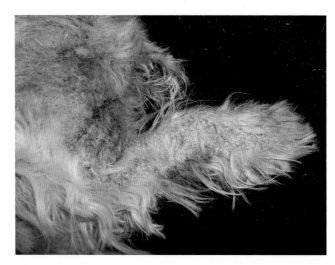

Figure D.2 Shows the right forelimb of an elderly West Highland White terrier. There is extensive alopecia, erythema and hyperpigmentation. The skin over the leg is covered in fine silvery white scale. Exfoliated scale is visible on the black rubber matting supporting the dog. This dog has adult onset generalised demodicosis.

Scale can be dry and readily separating from the skin surface, or greasy and forming loose cohesive layers. Dry scale is easy to sample with adhesive tape, while greasy scale will adhere to a clean glass slide. Scale is an obvious clinical sign in a wide range of skin disorders and can be a primary or a secondary feature. Scale is a very common secondary feature of chronic skin inflammation; for example, in dermatophytosis, allergic skin disease or bacterial pyoderma. Exfoliative dermatitis is the most common cutaneous manifestation of leishmaniosis in the dog.

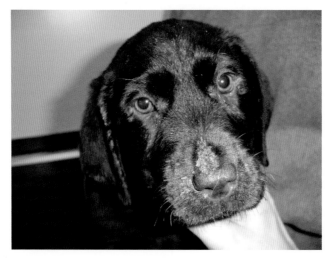

Figure D.3 Shows the face of an 8 week-old female Labrador Retriever puppy with a primary keratinisation disorder. The pup has a dull and lustreless coat from 1 week of age. Numerous clumps of greasy scale are noticed throughout the entire hair coat from 2 weeks of age and these have remained unchanged in appearance. There is no pruritus and the pup is bright and well. The other nine puppies in the litter have no skin lesions.

Crust is an accumulation of adherent dried material on the skin surface. Crust can contain dried blood, pus, applied medication, exudate and skin cells. There may also be matted hair, environmental debris and bacteria in the crust. Dark coloured crusts tend to contain a higher proportion of blood and usually reflect deeper pathology such as vasculitis or deep bacterial pyoderma. Crusts that are tightly adherent to the skin are more commonly associated with zinc responsive dermatosis and hepatocutaneous syndrome.

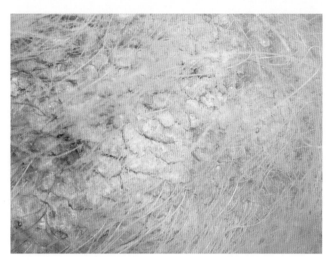

Figure D.4 Shows the skin over the lateral abdomen of a young Collie. There is generalised erythema and extensive thick pale-yellow crust formed of dried serum. The dog has a pruritic skin condition of approximately 11 months' duration and has received intermittent courses of oral prednisolone or oclacitinib. *Sarcoptes* mites were readily found on superficial skin scrapings from this area of skin.

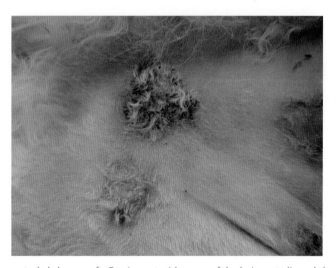

Figure D.5 Shows the ventral abdomen of a Persian cat with some of the hair coat clipped short. There is adherent crust around all of the nipples. The crust has been removed at the top right of the photograph and reveals an erythematous and eroded area. This cat has pemphigus foliaceus and the crust is largely composed of dried neutrophils and epidermal cells. The cat also has a large amount of caseous material in all of the nail beds.

History

A 5 year-old female neutered wire-haired Hungarian Vizsla is presented, as an emergency, with a 36-hour history of reluctance to stand, refusing her food and hyperventilation. The dog has been increasingly reluctant to exercise or play over the past few weeks. There are no other animals in the household and the dog is regularly dewormed. No routine vaccinations have been given since puppyhood.

Questions

1. Describe the abnormalities and pertinent normal features in Figures 21.1–21.4.
2. What differential diagnoses should be considered for this presentation?
3. What tests could you perform to make the diagnosis?

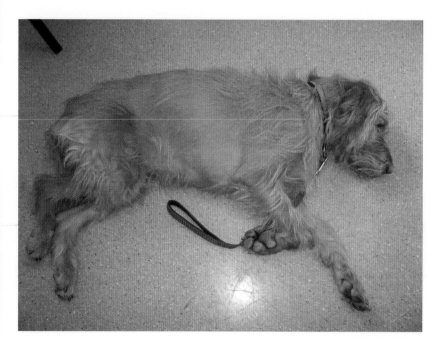

Figure 21.1

Small Animal Dermatology: What's Your Diagnosis? First Edition. Jane Coatesworth.
© 2019 John Wiley & Sons, Inc. Published 2019 by John Wiley & Sons, Inc.

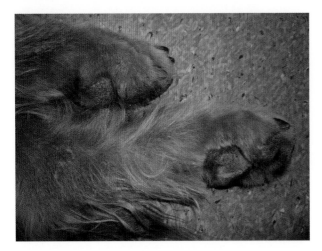

Figure 21.2

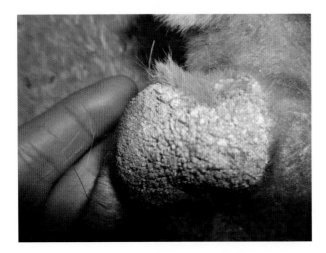

Figure 21.3

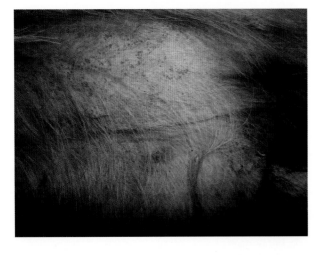

Figure 21.4

Answers

1. What the figures show

Figure 21.1 shows an inactive dog in pain, lying in lateral recumbency during the whole consultation. The dog is very reluctant to take any weight on the paws.

Figure 21.2 shows both front paws. There is marked erythema and swelling of the distal forelimbs and both front paws. Three large and tightly adherent crusts are visible on the medial aspect of the left fore. The pads are hyperkeratotic.

Figure 21.3 shows hyperkeratosis of the metacarpal pad of the left fore paw. The surrounding skin is markedly erythematous and swollen. All of the other foot pads and paws are similarly affected.

Figure 21.4 shows the groin. There is a large epithelial collarette, with a peeling epithelial edge and an erythematous centre, on the right of the picture and a smaller focus of crust and inflammation on the left. There are multiple epithelial collarettes and crusts over the body, including on the pinnae. The collarettes and crusts are up to 2 cm in diameter and span multiple hair follicles.

2. Differential diagnoses

Given the appearance of the skin lesions the following conditions should be considered:

Causes of hyperkeratotic footpads

- Pemphigus foliaceus (PF)
- Hypothyroidism
- Hepatocutaneous syndrome
- Distemper
- Idiopathic hyperkeratosis of specific breeds. This can affect the nasal planum and footpads of Springer Spaniels, or just the footpads in the Irish Terrier, Kromfohrlander and Dogue de Bordeaux.

Causes of widespread pustules containing neutrophils

- Superficial bacterial pyoderma
- PF
- Pustular dermatophytosis
- Drug eruption

3. Appropriate diagnostic tests

Physical examination shows a very subdued dog, which is carried into the examination room and immediately lies down in lateral recumbency. The prescapular and popliteal lymph nodes are markedly enlarged.

Dermatological examination, in addition to changes shown in the photographs, shows a band of erythema and hyperkeratosis at the junction of the dorsal nasal planum and the haired skin. The feet feel hot and are very painful to touch.

Cytology. A stained impression smear from the moist under surface of a crust shows high numbers of neutrophils and intracytoplasmic cocci and some acantholytic cells. The presence of cocci inside the neutrophils suggests a bacterial skin infection. Low numbers of acantholytic cells are commonly found in bacterial pyoderma. However, the clinical findings of large epithelial collarettes and crusts, including on the ear pinnae, are more suggestive of PF than bacterial infection. Secondary bacterial pyoderma is common in many skin diseases and is likely to be complicating the clinical picture here.

Skin biopsies are taken from lesional skin on the lateral thorax and one fore limb. Histology, from both sites, shows a hyperplastic epidermis with a prominent keratin layer. There are intra-epidermal and subcorneal pustules. Numerous acantholytic keratinocytes are present in the pustules. There is an inflammatory reaction in the superficial part of the dermis, characterised by the presence of neutrophils and a few eosinophils and macrophages. Periodic acid Schiff (PAS) staining shows no fungal elements in the examined sections. These changes are consistent with PF.

Diagnosis

Pemphigus foliaceus.

Treatment

The dog is given immediate analgesia with tramadol at $3\,\text{mg}\,\text{kg}^{-1}$ q 8 h and paracetamol at $10\,\text{mg}\,\text{kg}^{-1}$ q 12 h. Non-steroidal anti-inflammatories are avoided, as the dog is likely to need glucocorticoids very soon. Oral cephalexin is given, at $17\,\text{mg}\,\text{kg}^{-1}$ q 12 h, to address the bacterial pyoderma.

Prednisolone, at $2\,\text{mg}\,\text{kg}^{-1}$ once daily in the morning with food, is started once the diagnosis is made.

Three weeks later. The owner reports a brighter dog, but still subdued in comparison to her normal demeanour. There is a moderately increased thirst and appetite and also frequent panting. No new skin lesions have appeared. There are multifocal dry crusted areas over the trunk and concave aspects of the pinnae. The weight bearing aspects of the pads are much smoother, but there is persistent hyperkeratosis on the non-weight bearing pad margins. The degree of foot swelling is significantly reduced and the dog is walking but not wanting to exercise. The feet are still tender to touch. Prednisolone is continued at $2\,\text{mg}\,\text{kg}^{-1}$ once daily by mouth. The owner is asked to bathe the dog weekly with a chlorhexidine based shampoo to remove crust and scale, and to reduce the risk of recurrent secondary bacterial skin infection.

A further 3 weeks later. The dog is bright and active, with normal behaviour. There has been a single episode of vomiting and no new skin lesions. There are multifocal alopecic and hyperpigmented macules and patches at the sites of previous lesions. All of the footpads show a reduced degree of hyperkeratosis. The owner is asked to taper the dose of prednisolone by giving 2 and $1\,\text{mg}\,\text{kg}^{-1}$ on alternate days for 2 weeks, then 2 and $0.5\,\text{mg}\,\text{kg}^{-1}$ on alternate days for 2 weeks.

Four weeks later. Early hair regrowth is present at the sites of previous lesions and no new lesions have occurred. The dog is well, with no apparent adverse effects from the medication. The owner is asked to reduce the dose of prednisolone to $2\,\text{mg}\,\text{kg}^{-1}$ on alternate days for 2 weeks, then $1\,\text{mg}\,\text{kg}^{-1}$ on alternate days for 2 weeks.

A further 4 weeks later. There are no skin lesions and the dog is well. Prednisolone is reduced to $0.5\,\text{mg}\,\text{kg}^{-1}$ every other day for 2 weeks, then discontinued.

Prognosis

Good, with response to appropriate treatment and tolerance of the medication. There is no relapse in this case after 3 years of follow up.

Discussion

Keratinocytes are normally attached to each other by desmosomes at numerous points on their cell margins. This robust intercellular adhesion allows normal skin to be a resilient and cohesive structure, despite the frequent stretching and shearing forces placed upon it. Desmocollin-1 is a structural component of desmosomes and is the major target of auto-antibodies in canine PF. Intercellular adhesion is lost in focal areas of the middle layers of the epidermis – the stratum spinosum or stratum granulosum. Neutrophils move into the intra-epidermal clefts to form pustules. Keratinocytes that have lost their attachments to adjacent cells are called acantholytic. Acantholytic keratinocytes are large cells with a rounded outline, a clearly defined central nucleus and a dark blue cytoplasm. They can often be found in cytology samples from pustules. Finding acantholytic keratinocytes is not specific for PF, but they are much more commonly seen in PF than in superficial bacterial pyoderma or in pustular dermatophytosis. The presence of rafts of acantholytic cells, rather than single cells, also occurs more commonly in PF.

Cases of PF benefit from a rapid diagnosis and early rigorous treatment to put the disease into remission. When there is complete remission the medication can be slowly tapered. A proportion of cases, like this one, will remain in remission after treatment is discontinued. The cases where clinical signs recur are likely to need long term therapy. It is important to adequately inform owners of how to identify any early signs of recurrence and the importance of reporting this. Relapses can be more challenging to treat than the initial presentation and need early active intervention with appropriate medication when they occur.

Approximately half of cases of PF will respond to prednisolone alone. The other half will need adjunctive treatment, such as azathioprine, alongside the prednisolone to put the disease into remission.

PF can occur after exposure to drugs and takes two different forms. Drug-induced PF continues to have active pathology after the inciting drug is withdrawn and needs immunosuppressive treatment. In contrast, a PF-like drug reaction will resolve spontaneously once the inciting drug is withdrawn. Drugs that have been associated with cases of PF include oral antibiotics, such as cephalexin and potentiated sulfonamides, and topical flea and flea/tick products such as dinotefuran/pyriproxyfen/permethrin (Vectra 3D), fipronil/amitraz/S-methoprene (Certifect), and metaflumizone/amitraz (Promeris).

Further reading

Bizikova, P., Dean, G.A., Hashimoto, T., and Olivry, T. (2012). Cloning and establishment of canine desmocollin-1 as a major autoantigen in canine pemphigus foliaceus. *Veterinary Immunology and Immunopathology* 149: 197–207.

Bizikova, P., Linder, K.E., and Olivry, T. (2014). Fipronil-amitraz-S-methoprene-triggered pemphigus foliaceus in 21 dogs: clinical, histological and immunological characteristics. *Veterinary Dermatology* 25: 103–111.

Bizikova, P., Moriello, K.A., Linder, K.E., and Sauber, L. (2015). Dinotefuran/pyriproxyfen/permethrin pemphigus-like drug reaction in three dogs. *Veterinary Dermatology* 26: 206–208.

Kuhl, K.A., Shofer, F.S., and Goldschmidt, M.H. (1994). Comparative histopathology of pemphigus foliaceus and superficial folliculitis in the dog. *Veterinary Pathology* 31: 19–27.

Oberkirchner, U., Linder, K.E., Dunston, S. et al. (2011). Metaflumizone-amitraz (Promeris)-associated pustular acantholytic dermatitis in 22 dogs: evidence suggests contact drug-triggered pemphigus foliaceus. *Veterinary Dermatology* 22: 436–448.

Olivry, T. (2004). Prolonged remission after immunosuppressive therapy in six dogs with pemphigus foliaceus. *Veterinary Dermatology* 15: 245–252.

History

A 3 year-old female neutered Japanese Akita presents with a 6-month history of progressive hair loss. Loss of hair was first noticed on the legs, rump and perineum. Some hair has subsequently regrown in these areas. The owner reports that the head, neck and shoulders are the most recently affected areas. Although the owner has found a large volume of hair in the house, and the dog's coat has a much reduced appearance, they have never seen any bald areas of skin. The dog has not shown any pruritic behaviour in the last 6 months, and is bright and well. The other dog in the household is unaffected and the owners have no skin lesions.

Questions

1. Describe the abnormalities and pertinent normal features in Figures 22.1–22.3.
2. What differential diagnoses should be considered for this presentation?
3. What tests could you perform to make the diagnosis?

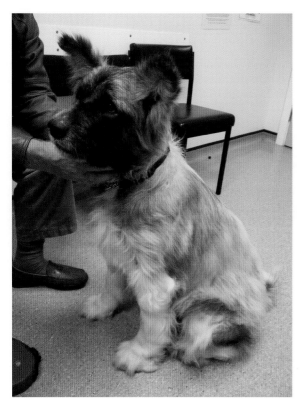

Figure 22.1

Small Animal Dermatology: What's Your Diagnosis? First Edition. Jane Coatesworth.
© 2019 John Wiley & Sons, Inc. Published 2019 by John Wiley & Sons, Inc.

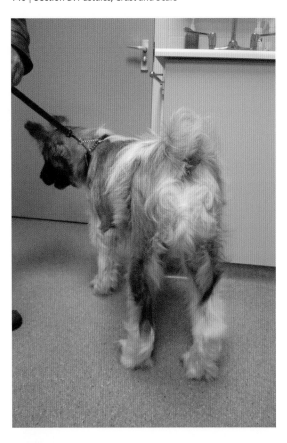

Figure 22.2

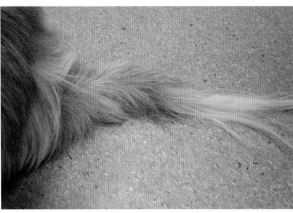

Figure 22.3

Answers

1. What the figures show

Figure 22.1 shows the dog from the left. There is significant thinning of the hair coat over the neck and trunk. The soft undercoat is largely absent, with only a proportion of the guard hairs remaining and resulting in a very atypical appearance for this breed. The hair coat is dull, dry and lustreless in appearance. The fore limbs, paws and ears are relatively unaffected.

Figure 22.2 shows the dog from behind. There is a marked reduction in the amount of secondary hair coat over the hind limbs and tail. The left hock has only overlying guard hairs, in contrast to the right hock that retains a secondary hair coat.

Figure 22.3 shows the sparsely haired tail. There is almost complete absence of the soft and voluminous secondary hair coat, resulting in a thin and atypical tail shape for this breed.

2. **Differential diagnoses**

   Given the appearance of the skin lesions the following conditions should be considered:

   - Sebaceous adenitis (SA)
   - Dermatophytosis. This condition is a cause of folliculitis, frequently presents with follicular casts and is usually non pruritic. However, discrete patches of hair loss would be more likely than the diffuse hypotrichosis seen in this case.
   - Demodicosis. The comment as for dermatophytosis is applicable.

3. **Appropriate diagnostic tests**

   General *physical examination* is unremarkable. Dermatological examination shows very numerous small clumps of hairs encased by follicular casts. These have a rigid feel on palpation and the hairs are easily epilated.

   Trichogram. Hair plucks, from the trunk and face, show follicular casts surrounding the hair shafts of a large proportion of hairs. The presence of follicular casts is a common and prominent feature of SA. They are also associated with follicular demodicosis (*Demodex canis*), and can be seen with dermatophytosis, which is another potential cause of follicular inflammation. No *Demodex* mites or fungal elements are seen.

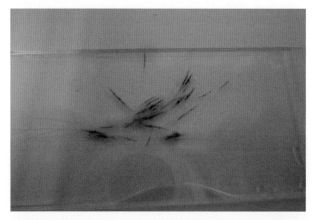

Figure 22.4 Shows some hairs plucked from the lateral thigh. The hairs are mounted in liquid paraffin under a glass cover slip. The root ends of small clumps of hair are bound together with dark coloured follicular casts.

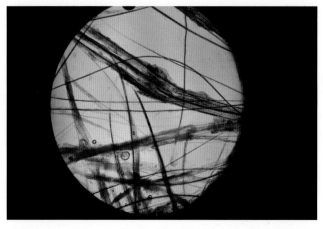

Figure 22.5 Shows a trichogram at ×400 magnification. The image is taken through the microscope, with the condenser partially lowered to increase contrast. A high proportion of the hair shafts are surrounded by follicular casts. Groups of two to seven hairs frequently lie in parallel and are joined into a firm mat by the surrounding cuffs of keratin. A group of three such hairs is seen here. The follicular casts extend from the hair bulb and encase from one-third to one-half of the length of the hair shafts.

Skin scrapes. Deep skin scrapes, down to capillary ooze, show no *Demodex* mites. Although *Demodex* are commonly found on hair plucks from affected dogs, negative deep skin scrapes are needed to exclude a diagnosis of follicular demodicosis.

Skin biopsies. Two full thickness skin biopsies are taken from the trunk, using local anaesthesia and a 6-mm biopsy punch. Histopathology shows a complete absence of sebaceous glands and there is no visible inflammatory reaction. The hair follicles contain a marked orthokeratotic hyperkeratosis. It is helpful to give the histopathologist a differential diagnosis of SA as it is more difficult to appreciate the absence, rather than the presence, of sebaceous glands.

Diagnosis

Sebaceous adenitis (SA).

Treatment

The dog is given oral ciclosporin, at 5 mg kg^{-1} once daily.

Options for topical therapy are discussed with the owner, who feels that the application of baby oil skin soaks would not be practical. They are happy to undertake daily spraying of the affected areas, with propylene glycol diluted 50 : 50 in water and occasional bathing with a sulfur and salicylic acid (keratolytic) shampoo.

Two months later there is early hair regrowth over the body. The dog is tolerating the ciclosporin well. Topical treatment has been sporadic and the hair coat feels dry and brittle. The dog appears comfortable and shows no signs of pruritus. The case is lost to further follow up.

Prognosis

SA is a largely cosmetic disease, and is usually only pruritic when complicated by secondary bacterial pyoderma. Most dogs respond to treatment, but regular ongoing treatment is required. The current therapies of choice are either labour intensive (topical treatment) or costly (ciclosporin), and best results usually occur with a combination of the two. The prognosis is often dependent on the time, facilities, funds and motivation available to an owner.

Discussion

The pathogenesis of SA is unknown, but the targeted inflammation and subsequent destruction of sebaceous glands is likely to be immune mediated. The condition is thought to involve T cell mediated inflammation of the sebaceous glands. Studies have shown no correlation between the historical duration of disease and the degree of sebaceous gland destruction. Histopathology can show a nodular inflammatory reaction at the level of the sebaceous glands, which is granulomatous to pyogranulomatous.

SA has a higher incidence in certain breeds, compared to the general dog population, suggesting a genetic influence. The disease is well recognised in the Standard Poodle, Samoyed, Hungarian Vizsla, English Springer spaniel, Hovawart, Havanese, Chow Chow and the Japanese Akita. The mode of inheritance in the Akita and the Standard Poodle is thought to be autosomal recessive. A wide range of other breeds and their crosses can be affected. The author has seen the condition in a number of Labradoodles. SA has a somewhat different clinical presentation between the breeds. The condition can present as large exfoliative sheets of skin cells restricted to the concave aspects of the pinnae and/or the ear canals.

SA is generally a non-pruritic condition, as in this case. However, dogs with SA are predisposed to secondary bacterial pyoderma, which can cause pruritus.

Topical therapy is helpful to soften and remove the scale and follicular casts, it also lubricates and conditions the hair coat. A number of topical treatment protocols are available. They involve a combination of washing the dog in a keratolytic shampoo, skin soaks in baby oil or calendula oil for 1–2 hours, and regular spraying with 50–70% propylene glycol in water. Topical treatment alone, or topical treatment in combination with ciclosporin, has been shown to reduce scaling more effectively than ciclosporin alone.

Ciclosporin is a helpful therapy for SA. Benefits are likely to occur from a combination of actions. These include the inhibition of T cell mediated inflammation, the induction of anagen to improve the quantity and quality of the hair coat, the induction of anagen to shift accumulated keratin from the hair follicle and the regeneration of sebaceous glands. Adverse effects of ciclosporin include vomiting and diarrhoea, in 25 and 15% of patients, respectively. These effects are usually transient and mild. Approximately 1% of dogs will develop gingival hyperplasia, which normally resolves with dose reduction or stopping ciclosporin therapy.

A good response to topical and/or ciclosporin therapy is usually seen after about 4 months. The treatment frequency can be tapered to achieve the best balance between a practical and affordable program for the client and a good outcome for the dog. Care needs to be taken in interpreting a response to treatment, as like many immune mediated diseases SA has a tendency to wax and wane in activity.

Other treatment options for SA include tetracycline/niacinamide, and essential fatty acid supplementation. Synthetic retinoids have variable efficacy in treating SA. Retinoids are a more expensive option than ciclosporin, and are currently difficult to obtain for veterinary use in the UK. Oral vitamin A has been used as an economical alternative to retinoids, associated with a reduced number of adverse effects, but the efficacy of treatment is variable and there is a lack of good evidence.

Further reading

Lortz, J., Favrot, C., Mecklenburg, L. et al. (2010). A multicentre placebo-controlled clinical trial on the efficacy of oral ciclosporin A and the treatment of canine idiopathic sebaceous adenitis in comparison with conventional topical treatment. *Veterinary Dermatology* 21: 593–601.

Reichler, I.M., Hauser, B., Schiller, I. et al. (2001). Sebaceous adenitis in the Akita: clinical observations, histopathology and heredity. *Veterinary Dermatology* 12: 243–253.

Steffan, J., Favrot, C., and Mueller, R. (2006). A systematic review and meta-analysis of the efficacy and safety of cyclosporin for the treatment of atopic dermatitis in dogs. *Veterinary Dermatology* 17: 3–16.

History

A 2 year-old female neutered Boxer presents with a 2-month history of 'dandruff'. The owner has tried to comb out the excess scale from the hair coat, but the problem rapidly returns. The dog shows no apparent signs of ill health or pruritus and has a regular vaccination and deworming programme. A spot-on product containing fipronil is applied monthly for flea control. There are no other pets in the household, but the dog has regular contact with other dogs by spending the day with a pet sitter three times each week. Two people in the family have had itchy skin lesions during the past month.

Questions

1. Describe the abnormalities and pertinent normal features in Figure 23.1.
2. What differential diagnoses should be considered for this presentation?
3. What tests could you perform to make the diagnosis?

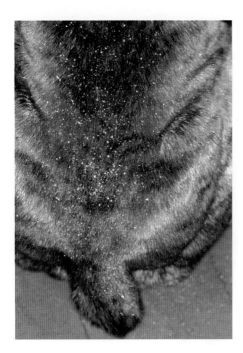

Figure 23.1

Small Animal Dermatology: What's Your Diagnosis? First Edition. Jane Coatesworth.
© 2019 John Wiley & Sons, Inc. Published 2019 by John Wiley & Sons, Inc.

Answers

1. What the figures show

Figure 23.1 shows the caudal dorsum and docked tail. There is a large amount of white scale and a few loose hairs on the hair coat. The individual scales are variable in size. The coat is glossy and in good condition, with no alopecia.

2. Differential diagnoses

Given the appearance of the skin lesions the following conditions should be considered:

- Cheyletiellosis.
- A cornification disorder, such as ichthyosis or primary seborrhoea. A cornification disorder is unlikely as the condition only started 2 months ago, and the dog had a normal and good quality coat for at least 2 years before the onset of clinical signs. The Boxer is not a predisposed breed for any of the recognised cornification disorders, but they can occasionally arise in an individual of any breed.

3. Appropriate diagnostic tests

Cytology. Samples are taken using a flea comb and adhesive tape strips. Samples of the dorsal scale are dislodged onto a piece of paper, collected onto a glass slide, mounted in liquid paraffin and covered with a glass cover slip.

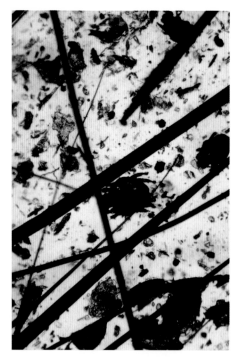

Figure 23.2 Shows an image from a coat brushing, mounted in liquid paraffin and viewed under the microscope with ×40 magnification. There is a large adult *Cheyletiella* mite in the centre, and a number of small juvenile mites at the periphery. A large egg is attached to a hair shaft at the bottom of the image. Surface living mites are typically fast moving and need to be mounted under a cover slip, or on acetate tape, to restrain them for identification.

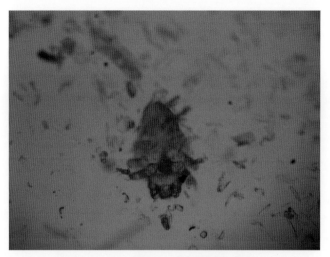

Figure 23.3 Shows detail from an acetate tape strip preparation. There is a *Cheyletiella* mite, seen in detail with ×100 magnification. The legs extend out beyond the outline of the body. The characteristic large curved hooks on the accessory mouthparts are visible at the bottom of the image.

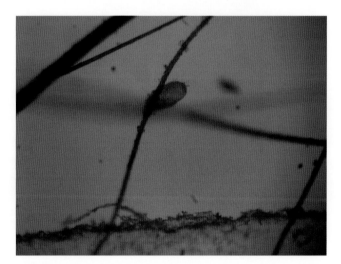

Figure 23.4 Shows detail from an acetate tape strip preparation, seen in detail with ×100 magnification. There is a *Cheyletiella* egg individually bound to a hair shaft by fine threads. The egg is approximately 0.25 mm long and elongated, and would be bound to the hair shaft just above the skin surface. *Cheyletiella* eggs are smaller than louse eggs (nits).

Diagnosis

Cheyletiellosis, with likely zoonotic spread to members of the family.

Treatment

The dog is sprayed all over, with a 0.25% w/v fipronil spray, every 3 weeks on three occasions. The house is sprayed with an environmental insecticidal spray containing permethrin, piperonyl butoxide and pyriproxyfen.

The pet sitter is informed of the diagnosis and referred to their local vet for suitable advice. The dog is kept away from the pet sitter until the infestation has cleared.

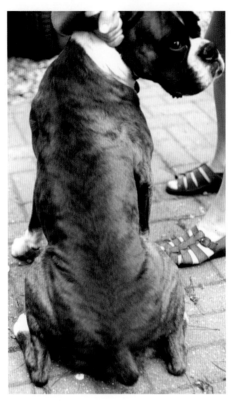

Figure 23.5 Shows the dog 2 months after the start of treatment. There is no visible scale and the hair coat is in good condition.

Prognosis

Good, if the *Cheyletiella* infestation can be successfully controlled.

Discussion

The 'dandruff' visible over the dorsal trunk in this case is comprised of a mixture of excess skin scale, *Cheyletiella* mites and mite eggs. *Cheyletiella* are large mites, up to 0.4 mm in length. Their visibility to the naked eye gives rise to the colloquial name 'walking dandruff'. Macroscopically, the mites are most evident when the skin debris is examined against a dark background. Diagnosis can be more challenging in cats with pruritus and excessive grooming, as they may remove the mites, eggs and skin scale from the coat. Faecal flotation can be useful in these cases to identify ingested *Cheyletiella* eggs and/or mites.

The dog in this case has high numbers of mites but no apparent pruritus. Affected individuals have very variable clinical signs. Clinical signs can range from no pruritus and a normal skin appearance, to severe self-excoriation and generalised erythema. The spectrum of clinical signs may be associated with the degree of hypersensitivity response mounted by the host towards mite allergens. In this case, it is likely that all of the four family members and the dog were bitten by the mites, but that only the two people with pruritic papules mounted a hypersensitivity response. Interestingly, the family member who regularly combed the scale out of the dog's coat had no clinical signs, despite the likelihood of regular exposure to mites. *Cheyletiella yasguri*, the species normally found on dogs, is not very host specific and will readily feed on people, rabbits and cats.

Cheyletiella mites feed on surface skin debris. They also use their mouthparts to pierce the epidermis and feed on tissue fluids. Female mites lay large eggs and attach them with slender fibres to individual hairs. The six-legged larvae emerges from the egg and progressively moults to become an eight-legged nymph and then an adult. The whole lifecycle takes place on the host. Adult female mites can survive for up to 10 days in the environment at average temperatures and longer if it is cool. The survival time off the host, as well as the mobility of the mites, makes treatment of the environment an important component in controlling an infestation.

Treatment is successful in this case with fipronil spray. Fipronil spray is likely to reach higher concentrations at the affected skin surface than fipronil spot-on, which the dog is already receiving. *Cheyletiella* complete their lifecycle in 3–5 weeks, so spraying at 3-week intervals is likely to be effective. Fipronil is potentially toxic to rabbits. Other treatment options for an affected individual are lime sulfur dip, permethrin shampoo (not for cats or rabbits as potentially toxic) or selamectin spot-on.

Further reading

Chadwick, A. (1997). Use of a 0.25% fipronil pump spray formulation to treat canine cheyletiellosis. *Journal of Small Animal Practice* 38: 261–262.

Chailleux, N. and Paradis, M. (2002). Efficacy of selamectin in the treatment of naturally acquired cheyletiellosis in cats. *Canadian Veterinary Journal* 43: 767–770.

History

An 8 year-old male neutered Chihuahua × Jack Russell Terrier is presented because of sore feet and crusty skin. Clinical signs were first noticed 3 months ago with interdigital erythema and a dry appearance to the pads. Crusts appeared 1 month ago, on the skin around the lips, and over the hocks and paws. All of the lesions have progressed in extent and severity with time. The dog is in pain in the affected areas and resents handling, but does not show any pruritic behaviour. The owner feels the dog has become less active, less interactive and has developed a variable appetite over the past 2 months. Routine vaccinations and anthelmintics have been given on a regular basis.

Questions

1. Describe the abnormalities and pertinent normal features in Figures 24.1–24.4.
2. What differential diagnoses should be considered for this presentation?
3. What tests could you perform to make the diagnosis?

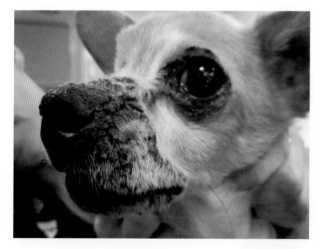

Figure 24.1

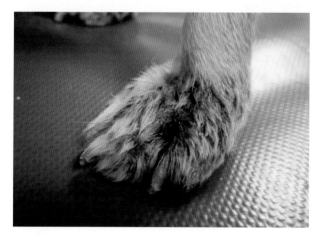

Figure 24.2

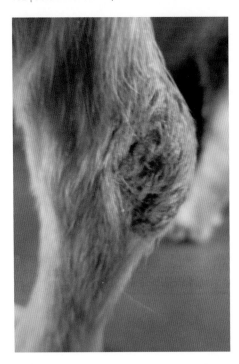

Figure 24.3

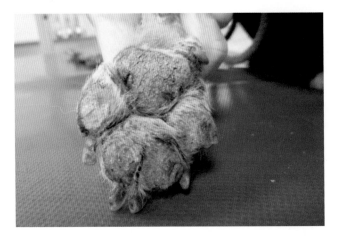

Figure 24.4

Answers

1. What the figures show

Figure 24.1 shows the left side of the face. There is thick adherent crust affecting a sharply demarcated area of the rostral muzzle and the periocular skin. The crusted areas are deeply fissured, with underlying erythema and erosion. These areas are painful. The dorsal and lateral margins of the nasal planum are also affected.

Figure 24.2 shows the lateral aspect of the left fore paw. There is severe and extensive erythema, exudation, crusting, eroded skin and matted hair. Note the normal appearance of the hair coat proximal to the metacarpophalangeal joints. The other fore paw is similarly affected.

Figure 24.3 shows the left lateral hock. There is thick, tightly adherent crust over the point of hock. Crusted areas are not alopecic. The hair coat is covered by, or incorporated into, the crust.

Figure 24.4 shows the palmar aspect of the left fore paw. There is marked hyperkeratosis of all of the footpads, with some cracking and fissuring. The long nails are typical of any chronic inflammatory pododermatitis and associated with increased blood supply to the nailbeds.

2. **Differential diagnoses**

Given the appearance of the skin lesions the following conditions should be considered:

Causes of hyperkeratosis of the footpads

- Hypothyroidism
- Pemphigus foliaceus
- Zinc responsive dermatosis
- Hepatocutaneous syndrome (HCS)
- Distemper
- Breed related hyperkeratosis (Dogue de Bordeaux, Irish Terrier, Kromfohrlander)

Causes of non-pruritic crusting of the hocks and muzzle

- Zinc responsive dermatosis
- HCS

3. **Appropriate diagnostic tests**

Haematology shows a raised white blood cell count of $24 \times 10^9 \, l^{-1}$ (6–$18 \times 10^9 \, l^{-1}$), and a neutrophilia of $21 \times 10^9 \, l^{-1}$ (4–$12 \times 10^9 \, l^{-1}$).

Serum biochemistry shows elevated alkaline phosphatase (ALP) $1488 \, iu \, l^{-1}$ (0–$150 \, iu \, l^{-1}$), alanine aminotransferase (ALT) $295 \, iu \, l^{-1}$ (0–$100 \, iu \, l^{-1}$), and bile acids $19 \, mmol \, l^{-1}$ (0–$15 \, mmol \, l^{-1}$). Increased ALP levels are found in hepatobiliary disease, especially with cholestasis, but are not specifically of hepatic origin. Elevated ALT is compatible with hepatocellular damage. There is a low urea of $2.3 \, mmol \, l^{-1}$ (2.8–$8.3 \, mmol \, l^{-1}$), probably reflecting the reduced conversion of ammonia to urea by an impaired liver.

An *adrenocorticotropic hormone (ACTH) stimulation test* is unremarkable and consistent with normal adrenal function.

Ultrasound examination of the abdomen shows that the liver is slightly small in size. The normal liver architecture is almost completely effaced by multiple hypoechoic regions of between 5 and 30 mm in diameter, which are surrounded by highly echogenic margins (see Figure 24.5). Only a small segment on the right side of the liver has a normal appearance. The portal blood flow is unremarkable. Examination of the rest of the abdomen, including the pancreas, is unremarkable.

Abdominal ultrasound, in cases of HCS, may show hepatic pathology or a pancreatic mass. The hepatic changes are generally either a vacuolar hepatopathy or cirrhosis, and the liver can be variable in size. A chronically cirrhotic liver appears small, with extensive fibrosis. Ascites may be present, along with reduced or reversed portal blood flow and acquired collateral circulation. Tissue for histopathology can be taken by ultrasound-guided liver biopsy or at exploratory laparotomy.

Skin cytology, using acetate tape strips, shows a moderate overgrowth of cocci and rods on the affected areas of the feet.

Skin biopsies. Full thickness skin biopsies are taken from the haired skin of the muzzle and from one paw. The biopsies show the characteristic 'red, white and blue' pattern of the epidermis in HCS, when stained with the usual haematoxylin and eosin (H&E) stains. This pattern represents 'red' parakeratotic hyperkeratosis (a dense layer of corneocytes with retained nuclei), a 'white' band of diffusely oedematous and necrotic keratinocytes and a 'blue' layer of hyperplastic basal and supra-basal keratinocytes. Areas of ulceration can be seen clinically and on histopathology. These arise from separation of the overlying crust along cleft lines in the central necrotic 'white' layer.

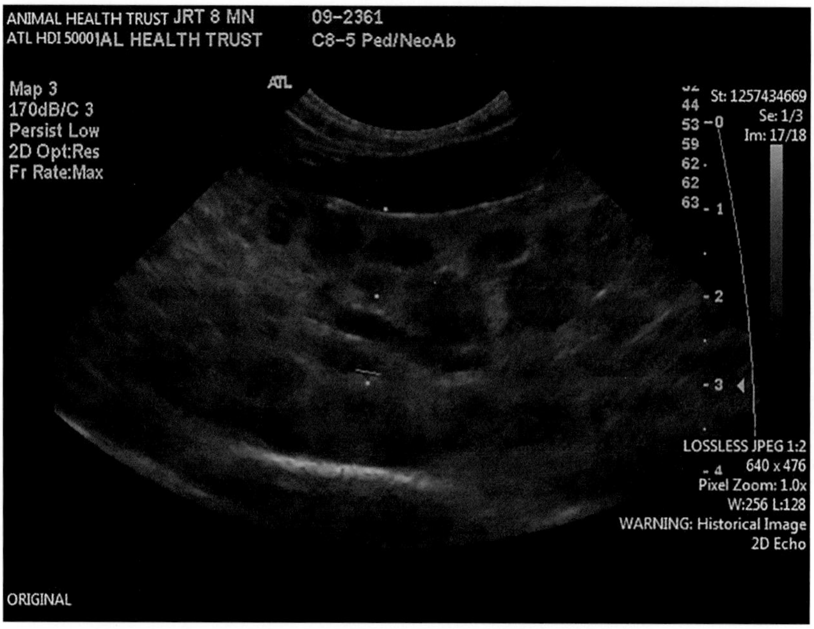

Figure 24.5 Shows an ultrasound image of the cranial abdomen. The liver has a 'honeycomb' or 'Swiss cheese' pattern, which is made of hypoechoic regions of variable sizes with hyperechoic margins.

Diagnosis

Hepatocutaneous syndrome. This condition is also referred to as superficial necrolytic dermatitis, metabolic epidermal necrosis, necrolytic migratory erythema and diabetic dermatopathy.

Treatment

No specific cause of the hepatopathy is identified in this case. A healthy liver has a significant degree of functional reserve, so clinical signs may only become apparent when extensive damage has already occurred and the original cause is no longer apparent. Effective treatment of an identified underlying cause can allow the liver to recover a degree of functionality and gives the best chance of longer term survival in this condition. The liver is unusual in having a significant capacity for regeneration, a process that is facilitated by feeding an optimal diet.

The diet is changed from regular dog food to a high quality commercial hepatic diet. This is supplemented with an additional source of readily digestible amino acids. The dog refuses to eat egg in any form, but is happy to eat soy protein powder mixed with a tinned hepatic diet formulation. The option of an intravenous infusion of amino acids is discussed with the owners. This treatment can give a temporary resolution of clinical signs, but lesions generally recur 1–2 weeks later and it is not effective in all dogs. The owners decline this option as they feel the dog would be unduly stressed by a day in the hospital.

A hydrogel spray, containing hypochlorous acid, is applied 2–3 times daily to the affected skin. After 1 week of treatment the bacterial overgrowth on the feet has resolved. The crusts are softer and more flexible and the dog appears to be more comfortable. This case has a mixed bacterial overgrowth, rather than a bacterial infection, on the affected skin of the feet. Hypochlorous acid is chosen here as it is non-toxic around the mouth and eyes, and can be used on broken skin. The gentle application of a keratolytic shampoo or moisturising ointment can reduce crust accumulation and skin fissuring and improve patient welfare.

Anti-inflammatory doses of prednisolone can temporarily improve the skin lesions, but will increase insulin resistance and may precipitate the onset of overt diabetes mellitus.

Prognosis

The prognosis can be good in the short term, as symptomatic treatment can significantly improve the quality of life.

The long term prognosis is poor if no specific underlying disease can be identified and treated. Patients generally survive months rather than years.

Discussion

HCS is an uncommon disease in the dog and is usually associated with an underlying hepatopathy. The analogous condition of necrolytic migratory erythema in humans is most often associated with an underlying glucagon – secreting pancreatic tumour, but this is a less common finding in the dog. The hepatopathy in canine cases is often idiopathic. Specific underlying causes for hepatopathy, which are identified in some cases, include hyperadrenocorticism, copper storage disease, diabetes mellitus, phenobarbitone toxicity and the ingestion of a mycotoxin. HCS is rare in the cat and identified underlying causes include hepatopathy and/or pancreatic carcinoma.

The pathophysiology of HCS is not well understood. An undefined metabolic dysfunction of the liver leads to nutritional deficiency and subsequent necrosis of skin cells. Abnormal glucagon balance and low amino acid levels appear to be part of the mechanism. The low levels may be due to increased hepatic metabolism of amino acids. Dogs with non-HCS associated hepatopathy tend to have elevated levels of amino acids due to reduced metabolism and clearance of proteins by the liver. Optimising the diet reduces the metabolic work load of the liver and may help with the nutritional deficiency at the level of the skin. The supplementation of zinc and essential fatty acids may also be helpful.

Intravenous infusions of amino acids can give temporary reversal of the clinical signs, supporting the nutritional deficiency theory. Infusions can be repeated at intervals as required. The addition of a concurrent lipid infusion was felt to increase the interval between the need for amino acid infusions in one case report. The interval increased from every 1.5 weeks to every 6.5 weeks on average, and the dog was maintained on the treatment for 2 years.

The condition often presents with thick adherent crusts, which are enmeshed in the hair coat. These crusts are partially comprised of a thick layer of dead skin cells. The crusts overlie, or are found adjacent to, areas of erythema, erosions and ulcers. They often have a bilaterally symmetrical distribution. Hyperkeratosis of the footpads seems to be a ubiquitous feature of the disease in the dog, often associated with fissures, exudation or haemorrhage and lameness. Soaking the pads in propylene glycol can have a helpful softening action. Lesions affect the skin around the mucocutaneous junctions, and are less commonly found on the pinnae, the pressure points and scrotum. These skin areas are mobile and the relatively rigid crusts are often cracked and painful. Topical therapy with emollient creams or ointments can afford some degree of symptomatic relief, if the application is not distressing for the patient and the product is not immediately licked off.

Bacterial overgrowths are a common finding when the integrity and barrier function of the skin is disrupted. They are generally managed by antimicrobial topical therapy, rather than with systemic antibiotics. Secondary bacterial, yeast or dermatophyte infections are also common findings with HCS. They need specific identification and treatment, as they contribute to poor patient welfare. It is important that the treatment given does not place undue metabolic stress on the liver.

The complete resolution of clinical signs after excision of a pancreatic glucagonoma is reported in a dog and in man. Glucagonomas often metastasise, so tumour staging is important to select appropriate surgical candidates.

Octreotide is a treatment option for dogs with glucagonoma-associated disease, when the primary tumour is not resectable or when metastasis has already occurred. Octreotide inhibits the release of glucagon, as well as inhibiting insulin and growth hormone release. Reduced appetite is the main adverse effect in the dog and the dose should be titrated to give a balance of positive effects.

Further reading

Bach, J.A. and Glasser, S.A. (2013). A case of necrolytic migratory erythema managed for 24 months with intravenous amino acid infusions. *Canadian Veterinary Journal* 54: 873–875.

Hill, P.B., Auxilia, S.T., Munro, E. et al. (2000). Resolution of skin lesions and long-term survival in a dog with superficial necrolytic dermatitis and liver cirrhosis. *Journal of Small Animal Practice* 41: 519–523.

Oberkirchner, U., Linder, K.E., Zadrozny, L., and Olivry, T. (2010). Successful treatment of canine necrolytic migratory erythema (superficial necrolytic dermatitis) due to metastatic glucagonoma with octreotide. *Veterinary Dermatology* 21: 510–516.

Outerbridge, C.A., Marks, S.L., and Rogers, Q.R. (2002). Plasma amino acid concentrations in 36 dogs with histologically confirmed superficial necrolytic dermatitis. *Veterinary Dermatology* (4): 177–186.

Torres, S., Caywood, D.D., O'Brien, T.D. et al. (1997). Resolution of superficial necrolytic dermatitis following excision of a glucagon secreting pancreatic neoplasm in a dog. *Journal of the American Animal Hospital Association* 33: 313–319.

History

A 12 year-old female neutered Jack Russell terrier presents with a 3-year history of mild to moderate pruritus and a progressively increasing degree of scaling. The scaling starts on the rostral muzzle and progresses caudally to the head and ears. The condition waxes and wanes in severity. The dog is a dedicated and skilled hunter and lives on a farm. The diet is a complete dry food, supplemented by self-caught wild rabbits and rodents. The owners have regularly seen fleas on the dog and occasionally apply a spot-on flea treatment. Routine vaccinations are given every year. The dog has free access to the farm during the day and sleeps in the kitchen overnight. The owners have no skin lesions, despite regular contact with the dog, and no other pets. A variety of treatments have been given over the years, including topical tea tree oil, four courses of oral antibiotics, oral methylprednisolone at 0.4 mg kg^{-1} every other day for 3 weeks, miconazole/chlorhexidine shampoo twice weekly for 6 weeks, chlorhexidine scrub twice weekly for 3 weeks and enilconazole rinse weekly for 6 weeks on two separate occasions. The owner reports that the only response to treatment was with glucocorticoids, which temporarily stopped the pruritus.

Questions

1. Describe the abnormalities and pertinent normal features in Figures 25.1 and 25.2.
2. What differential diagnoses should be considered for this presentation?
3. What tests could you perform to make the diagnosis?

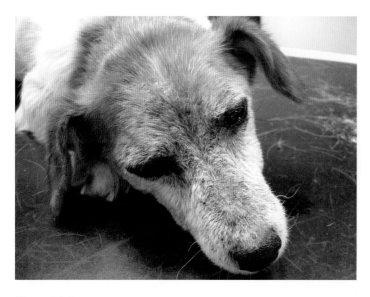

Figure 25.1

Small Animal Dermatology: What's Your Diagnosis? First Edition. Jane Coatesworth.
© 2019 John Wiley & Sons, Inc. Published 2019 by John Wiley & Sons, Inc.

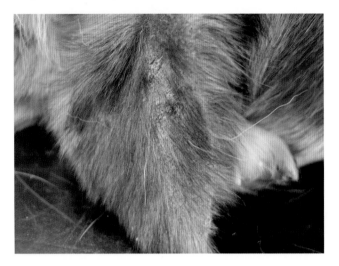

Figure 25.2

Answers

1. **What the figures show**

    Figure 25.1 shows the dog when sedated, with lubricant gel in both eyes. There is abundant thick grey scale around the eyes and over the top of the head. The rostral edge of the right pinna is alopecic and has a layer of thick adherent scale. There is an area of alopecia on the dorsal muzzle. The whiskers are sparse and misshapen. The skin of the head and ears is hyperpigmented with no erythema.

    Figure 25.2 shows the convex aspect of the right pinna. There is hypotrichosis, especially of the rostral part. A thick layer of grey scale covers the entire pinnal surface, but is partially obscured by the hair coat. There are linear excoriations at the top of the most alopecic area.

2. **Differential diagnoses**

    Given the appearance of the skin lesions the following conditions should be considered:

    - Dermatophytosis, particularly *Trichophyton mentagrophytes* or *Microsporum persicolor*.
    - Pemphigus foliaceus is considered due to the symmetrical facial distribution, the waxing and waning course of the disease, and the prominent scaling. However, this dog has no loss of pigment or ulceration and erosion of the nasal planum, which would be common findings in pemphigus foliaceus.
    - Bacterial skin infection is a common cause of secondary crust and scale, but this dog has shown no response to four separate courses of antibiotics. The dog has lesions on the pinna, which is an unusual location for bacterial pyoderma.

3. **Appropriate diagnostic tests**

    Wood's lamp. There is no fluorescence of hairs when the affected areas are illuminated by a Wood's lamp. This test is helpful when it shows a positive result. Only a proportion of *Microsporum canis* isolates fluoresce under ultraviolet light, so a negative result does not rule out dermatophytosis. The history of regular hunting, and the predominance of scale rather than alopecia, make *Trichophyton* or *M. persicolor* more likely than *M. canis* in this case.

    Cytology. Examination of skin scale and plucked hairs mounted in liquid paraffin does not show any fungal elements.

    Dermatophyte culture. Samples of scale and plucked hairs, from the head and the right pinna, are submitted to a laboratory for fungal culture.

    Skin biopsies are taken for histopathology from the affected skin of the head. Biopsies are taken with an 8 mm biopsy punch, using local anaesthesia and with the dog under sedation. The epidermis shows moderate to severe hyperkeratosis with areas of parakeratosis and inflammatory crust formation. The upper and mid-dermis show a few irregular areas of a moderate perivascular infiltrate of mixed inflammatory cells, mainly lymphocytes and plasma cells. Normal numbers of hair follicles are present and most are in anagen. Sebaceous glands are hypertrophied. Special staining with periodic acid Schiff shows small numbers of fungal hyphae present in the keratin crusts. No fungal hyphae are found in the hair shafts.

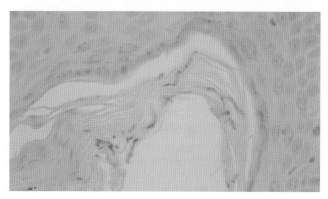

Figure 25.3 Shows a section of epidermis stained with periodic acid Schiff (PAS), from a skin biopsy of the head. There are purple-staining fungal hyphae in the hyperkeratotic layers of the stratum corneum.

Diagnosis
Dermatophytosis. Fungal culture confirmed the dermatophyte as *M. persicolor*.

Treatment
Oral itraconazole is given with food at 5 mg kg^{-1} once daily for 7 days, stopped for 7 days and then repeated. Haematology and serum biochemistry show no abnormalities in this older dog. Blood samples are taken before treatment with itraconazole and serum biochemistry is repeated after the first 4 weeks of treatment.

The head and neck are wiped with diluted lime sulfur dip. The solution is applied once a week with a cosmetic sponge and allowed to dry on the skin. The sponge ensures even and accurate application of solution to the skin and no free liquid running in an uncontrolled direction.

The owners are informed of the potentially contagious nature of dermatophytosis and given information on environmental and hand hygiene. *Microsporum persicolor* has a low zoonotic potential in comparison to *M. canis*. The dog sleeps in the kitchen overnight so cleaning efforts are focused on the kitchen and the dog bedding to reduce the number of spores in the environment. The owner vacuums to pick up loose skin scale, cleanses hard surfaces with a detergent to remove organic debris and then wipes down the clean surfaces with dilute household bleach. The bedding is washed twice weekly in the home washing machine at 30°C using the longest wash cycle.

The dog responds well to treatment, with progressive reduction of the excess scaling. Two negative dermatophyte cultures are obtained 4 weeks apart after a total of 12 weeks of treatment.

Prognosis
The prognosis is good for resolution of this infection. There is a risk of repeated infection given the lifestyle and hunting behaviour of this dog and the consequent risk of infection directly from small rodents, or indirectly from their habitats.

Discussion
Dermatophytes produce enzymes that allow them to utilise the dead keratin protein of skin, hair or nails as a source of nutrition. Different species of dermatophyte are adapted to particular species of animals or

to live in the soil. The fungal hyphae of *M. persicolor* invade the superficial layers of the stratum corneum and do not affect the hair shafts or nails. It is logical to think that the examination of skin scale will readily reveal fungal hyphae and/or spores in cases of *M. persicolor*. Unfortunately, such direct examinations are normally unrewarding, including in this case.

Microsporum persicolor is one of the less common dermatophytes to cause skin infection in the general dog population in the United Kingdom. There is a different incidence of the various dermatophytes in different geographical areas. *Microsporum persicolor* is more commonly isolated from dogs that have regular contact with rodents. Studies of small rodents in their wild habitats show that *M. persicolor* predominates in bank voles, that bank voles are frequently and often heavily infected with *M. persicolor* and that infections in bank voles may persist for several months. This dog had unrestricted and extensive access to a rural environment and was known to catch small rodents on a regular basis.

The dog in this case has a 3-year history of clinical signs and it is likely that infection has been present for this period. Other cases of *M. persicolor* are reported with durations of between 3 and 5 years. It may be that, in *M. persicolor* infection, the superficial layers of the stratum corneum are far enough removed from the host cell mediated immune response to make effective identification and clearance of the infection a difficult task. The absence of erythema seen in this case suggests that the immune system is not mounting a significant inflammatory response.

A review of 119 cases of *M. persicolor* showed lesions to be most frequent on the head (84.7%) and less frequent on the body and legs (11.1–23.6%). Alopecia and crusts were the most common lesions. Pruritus and scaling were more frequently seen in older dogs, and pruritus was more frequent after 1 month of infection. The excessive scaling in this case is likely to be due to an increased epidermal turnover rate triggered in response to the infection. The increased loss of surface skin scales helps to remove dermatophyte from the host, but contributes to contamination of the environment.

A breach in the integrity of the skin surface is necessary for the initial dermatophyte infection to take hold. This dog may have sustained accidental trauma while hunting or may have been scratched or bitten by a prey species. The history of frequent fleas may have contributed to microtrauma from flea bites, particularly from rabbit fleas that are active around the head.

The dog in this case had received a number of topical products with antifungal activity in the past. The products were administered for periods of 3 or 6 weeks, which may have been too short a period to see a response, especially when they were used without additional systemic treatment. Poor compliance may also have been an issue when treating the head area of this independently minded dog. Lime sulfur is chosen to treat this dog as it is quick and simple to apply and has good activity against fungal spores. The product does not need to be massaged into the skin and is left on the skin to dry. Topical enilconazole solution would fulfil these desirable criteria, but lime sulfur also has a keratolytic action and is helpful in removing the excess layers of skin scale in this case.

Further reading

Bond, R., Middleton, D.J., Scarff, D.H., and Lamport, A.I. (1992). Chronic dermatophytosis due to *Microsporum persicolor* infection in three dogs. *Journal of Small Animal Practice* 33: 571–576.

Bond, R. (2002). Canine dermatophytosis associated with *Trichophyton* species and *Microsporum persicolor*. *In Practice* 24: 388–395.

Bourdeau, P., Delage, A., Hubert, F. et al. (2014). *Microsporum persicolor* in the dog: a series of 119 cases. In: *Proceedings of the 27th ESVD/ECVD Congress, Salzburg, Austria*, September 2014, 167.

Carlotti, D. and Bensignor, E. (1999). Dermatophytosis due to *Microsporum persicolor* (13 cases) or *Microsporum gypseum* (20 cases) in dogs. *Veterinary Dermatology* 10: 17–27.

English, M.P. and Bayley, J.A. (1978). Dermatophytes in a population of bank voles and wood mice. *Mycopathologia* 66: 67–71.

History

A 6 year-old male neutered Domestic Shorthaired cat presents with a 4-week history of crusted lesions on the face and ears. The lesions have slowly increased in size over the weeks and the owner describes intermittent flicking of the ears.

Questions

1. Describe the abnormalities and pertinent normal features in Figures 26.1–26.4.
2. What differential diagnoses should be considered for this presentation?
3. What tests could you perform to make the diagnosis?

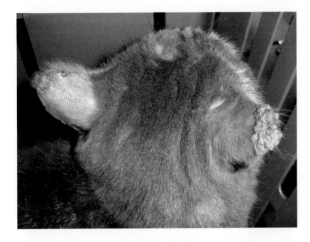

Figure 26.1

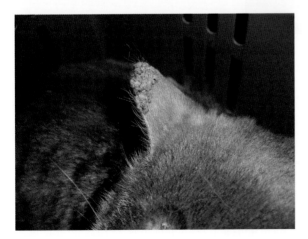

Figure 26.2

Small Animal Dermatology: What's Your Diagnosis? First Edition. Jane Coatesworth.
© 2019 John Wiley & Sons, Inc. Published 2019 by John Wiley & Sons, Inc.

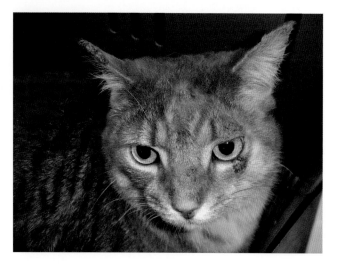

Figure 26.3

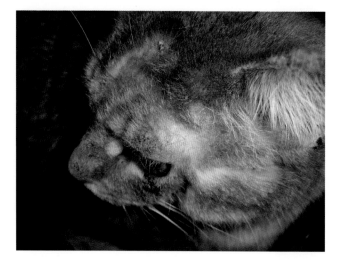

Figure 26.4

Answers

1. What the figures show

Figure 26.1 shows the back of the head. There are well demarcated crusted lesions on the tips of the pinnae and on the mid-forehead. The skin immediately adjacent to the crust is erythematous and swollen. There is hypotrichosis of the convex aspect of the left pinna.

Figure 26.2 shows a closer view of the right pinnal lesion. There is a sharp demarcation between the affected and normal skin. The pinnal tip is covered with thick adherent yellowish crust, interspersed with haemorrhagic crust.

Figure 26.3 shows the cat's face. There are erythematous and crusted lesions on the mid-forehead, bridge of the nose, pinnal tips, inside the left lateral pinnal margin and above and below the left eye. There is erosion of the nasal planum, especially on the left side of the nasal philtrum.

Figure 26.4 shows discrete crusted lesions on the mid-forehead, inside the left pinna, on the bridge of the nose, and above and below the left eye. The associated and well circumscribed erythema is most visible in the thinly haired area above the left eye.

2. **Differential diagnoses**

> Given the appearance of the skin lesions, the following conditions should be considered:

- Pemphigus foliaceus (PF)
- Dermatophytosis
- Notoedric mange
- Bacterial superficial pyoderma

3. **Appropriate diagnostic tests**

> *Cytology.* A section of crust is removed from one of the pinnae and from the face. The moist underside of the crust is touched onto a glass slide and stained with a modified Romanowsky stain (Rapi-Diff). Light microscopy under low (×40) and medium (×100) power shows non-degenerate neutrophils and numerous acantholytic keratinocytes.

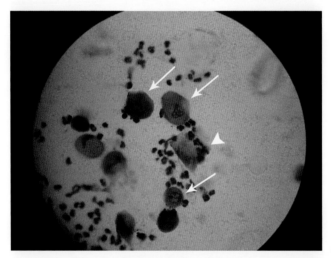

Figure 26.5 Shows a photomicrograph of a cytology preparation. The touch preparation was made from the moist underside of a facial crust. There are a number of rounded acantholytic keratinocytes with prominent nuclei (arrows). The rounded shape, and the visible nucleus, indicates their origin from deeper levels of the epidermis. In contrast, the thin angular cell with only a faint nuclear remnant (arrowhead) is a keratinocyte from a superficial level of the epidermis. Such cells are commonly encountered when examining acetate tape strip preparations. Numerous non-degenerative neutrophils make up the rest of the cell population. The neutrophils are small in comparison to the keratinocytes and have dark staining multi-lobed nuclei.

> *Skin biopsies* are taken, under general anaesthesia, from the facial lesions. They show mild to moderate irregular epidermal hyperplasia and subcorneal pustules containing non-degenerate neutrophils and acantholytic cells. There is a mixed superficial perivascular dermatitis. There is no evidence of bacteria, mites or dermatophytes and periodic acid Schiff (PAS) staining does not highlight any dermatophytes. These changes are consistent with a subcorneal pustular dermatitis, and PF.

Diagnosis

Pemphigus foliaceus (PF).

Treatment

Oral prednisolone is given at 2.6 mg kg^{-1} once daily.

Re-evaluations and final outcome

After 3 weeks of high dose oral prednisolone the lesions have substantially resolved. There is hypotrichosis at the previously crusted sites, no erythema and a few small crusts on the caudal pinnal margins. The dose of prednisolone is reduced by one-third every 2 weeks.

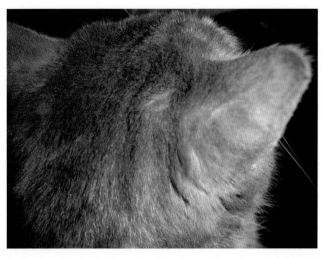

Figure 26.6 Shows the back of the head after 3 weeks of treatment. There is complete resolution of the mid-forehead and pinnal lesions. A few small crusts are palpable on the caudal pinnal margins.

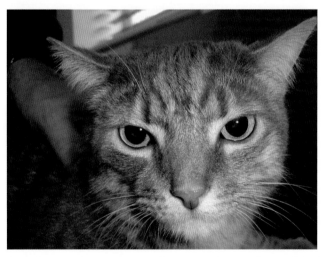

Figure 26.7 Shows the face after 3 weeks of treatment. There is complete resolution of the facial lesions, including the nasal ulceration and the crusting on the inner aspect of the left pinna.

Four weeks later there is complete resolution of the lesions. The dose of prednisolone is tapered, to 1 mg kg^{-1} every other day, over a further 4 weeks and then to 0.5 mg kg^{-1} every other day. After 3 weeks on this low dose, the cat was still lesion free and the prednisolone was discontinued.

Two months after stopping treatment crusted lesions recur on the caudal edge of the left pinna. Cytology shows non-degenerative neutrophils and acantholytic keratinocytes. Oral prednisolone is restarted at 2.6 mg^{-1} kg^{-1} day. The lesions resolve completely in 2 weeks and the prednisolone is tapered slowly, over 12 weeks, to 0.5 mg kg^{-1} every other day. The cat is maintained on this dose and has no recurrence of lesions over the subsequent 4 years. Serum biochemistry, haematology and urinalysis are monitored annually and there are no apparent adverse effects from the treatment.

Prognosis

Good with continued response to treatment and ongoing tolerance of the medication.

Discussion

PF is an autoimmune skin disease but the specific autoantigen and pathogenesis have not been characterised in the cat.

This case shows a typical lesion distribution involving the face and pinnae. A review of 57 cases showed head or face lesions in 78.9% of the cases and pinnal lesions in 68.4%. The lesions in this case were asymmetrical on the face, while the same review found a high proportion of cases to have symmetrical facial lesions. Purulent material in the claw folds, and lesions around the nipples, are common clinical signs in cats but were not features of this case.

There was a complete response to treatment in this case and relapse 2 months after stopping therapy. A proportion of cases of PF, in both cats and dogs, do not require long-term medication once they have gone into remission. The author attempts to take all patients off therapy after slowly tapering the immunosuppressive treatment. It is important to catch relapses early by ensuring that owners can recognise recurrent lesions and are motivated to report them. Recurrent disease can be more difficult to get into remission than the initial presentation and is best treated rigorously as soon as it occurs. Stopping therapy, in those cases that do not need it, minimises the potential harm of long-term drug treatment. This cat resents taking tablets but alternate day therapy is manageable for the owner.

Bacterial superficial pyoderma is a common cause of subcorneal pustular dermatitis, but was an unlikely diagnosis in this case. No bacteria were seen on cytology or histopathology. Cats are affected with bacterial pyoderma much less frequently than dogs, and the pinnal tips would be an unusual lesion site in either species. Bacterial pyoderma is generally secondary to another inciting cause and can complicate cases of PF.

Further reading

Griffin, C.E. (1991). Recognising and treating pemphigus foliaceus in cats. *Veterinary Medicine* 86: 513–516.

Preziosi, D.E., Goldschmidt, M.H., Greek, J.S. et al. (2003). Feline pemphigus foliaceus: a retrospective analysis of 57 cases. *Veterinary Dermatology* 14: 313–321.

History

A 1-year-old male neutered Siberian Husky is presented with a history of lethargy and pruritus. The dog was acquired from a rescue centre 4 months ago with a diagnosis of sarcoptic mange. The dog has had three previous owners. The current owners gave the dog four washes with amitraz solution at weekly intervals, to follow on from the three weekly washes at the rescue centre. At the time of acquisition, the dog was underweight, moderately pruritic, had persistent diarrhoea and had difficulty walking on severely swollen feet. The referring veterinary surgeon gave cephalexin at 22 mg kg^{-1} every 12 h for 6 weeks and the skin and gut signs resolved. Skin signs returned 6 weeks later with chewing of the tail base, licking of the abdomen and biting of the legs and feet. Prednisolone was dispensed at 0.5 mg^{-1} kg^{-1} day for 10 days, and increased to 1 mg^{-1} kg^{-1} day for 10 days when the pruritus was unresponsive. Facial lesions, severe self-excoriation and lethargy are features of the past 2 weeks. The dog is lethargic, has a peripheral lymphadenopathy and has worn an Elizabethan collar for the last 2 weeks to reduce self-trauma.

Questions

1. Describe the abnormalities and pertinent normal features in Figures 27.1–27.6.
2. What differential diagnoses should be considered for this presentation?
3. What tests could you perform to make the diagnosis?

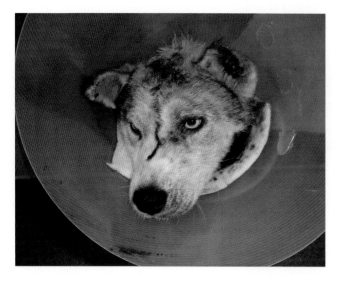

Figure 27.1

Small Animal Dermatology: What's Your Diagnosis? First Edition. Jane Coatesworth.
© 2019 John Wiley & Sons, Inc. Published 2019 by John Wiley & Sons, Inc.

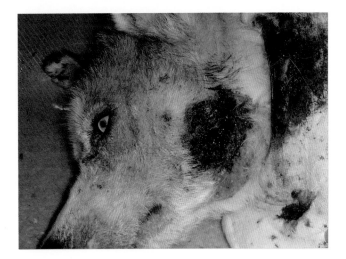

Figure 27.2

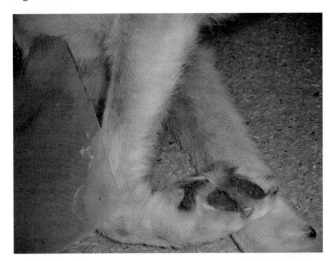

Figure 27.3

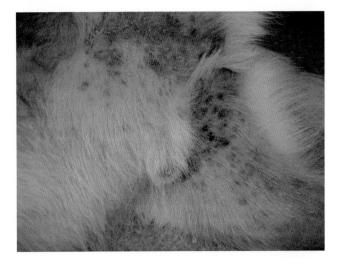

Figure 27.4

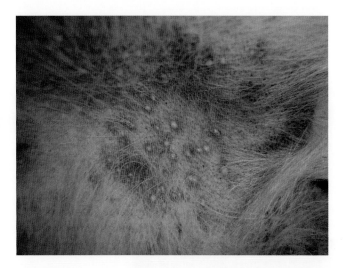

Figure 27.5

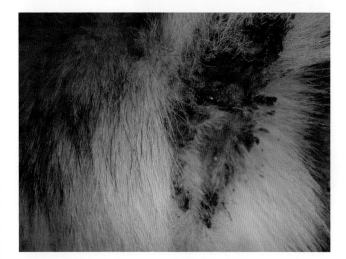

Figure 27.6

Answers

1. What the figures show

Figure 27.1 shows the dog at presentation, wearing an Elizabethan collar. There are ulcerated lesions with overlying crust between the ears and on the distal pinnae. Haemorrhagic exudate has run down between the eyes and dried onto the hair coat.

Figure 27.2 shows the left lateral face. The dog is lethargic. There is a large ulcerated lesion, partially covered in haemorrhagic crust on the left face. The skin is diffusely and intensely erythematous. The exudate-soaked gauze around the dog's neck has been reflected back to show the lesions.

Figure 27.3 shows both fore limbs. There is hypotrichosis and diffuse erythema. Follicular casts are seen around the nail beds.

Figure 27.4 shows the groin and right medial thigh. There are multiple erythematous papules and pustules.

Figure 27.5 shows a closer view of the groin. The prominent follicular pustules are round, have a surrounding erythematous margin and are greenish yellow in colour. The pustules are interspersed with black coloured comedones, particularly on the right side of the image.

Figure 27.6 shows the perineum. There is alopecia, erythema, crusting and large follicular pustules around the anus and on the proximal part of the ventral tail.

2. Differential diagnoses

Given the appearance of the skin lesions the following conditions should be considered:

- Bacterial folliculitis
- Demodicosis
- *Sarcoptes* infestation. The history and clinical signs are not typical, but the dog has a recent diagnosis of sarcoptic mange and a significant level of pruritus.

3. Appropriate diagnostic tests

Hair plucks from around the nail beds, and deep skin scrapes from the lateral left hind limb show high numbers of *Demodex* mites in all life stages.

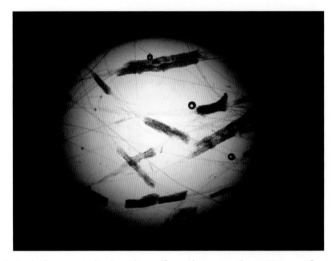

Figure 27.7 Shows a hair pluck, mounted in liquid paraffin and examined at ×40 magnification under the microscope. There are numerous follicular casts cuffing the hair shafts.

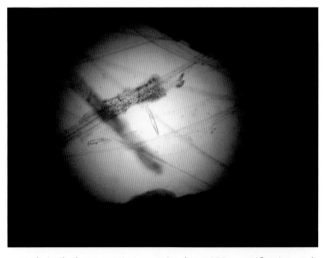

Figure 27.8 Shows the same hair pluck preparation, examined at ×100 magnification under the microscope. *Demodex* mites, in various life stages, are visible below and on the right side of the follicular cast.

Superficial skin scrapes show no *Sarcoptes* mites

Pustule cytology shows *Demodex* mites and high numbers of degenerative neutrophils with intracytoplasmic cocci.

Diagnosis

Juvenile-onset generalised demodicosis, with bacterial folliculitis.

Treatment

The corticosteroids are tapered over 5 days and discontinued. Cephalexin is given at 22 mg kg^{-1} every 12 h. Topical imidacloprid/moxidectin is dispensed for application every week, along with a chlorhexidine-based shampoo for weekly bathing.

Re-evaluations and final outcome

Three weeks later the dog is brighter and more active. The level of pruritus has reduced to a moderate level, allowing removal of the Elizabethan collar. There is intense erythema and partial alopecia of the face, limbs and ventrum. Cephalexin, chlorhexidine bathing and weekly imidacloprid/moxidectin are continued. The hair coat is clipped to a short length to facilitate topical therapy and easy assessment of the skin lesions.

Three weeks later there is no change in the clinical signs or the level of pruritus. Moderate to high numbers of *Demodex* in all life stages are found on skin scraping. The areas of previously broken skin surface have healed. Treatment is changed to weekly bathing in benzoyl peroxide shampoo, followed by amitraz dips of the whole dog at a 1 : 100 dilution (0.05%). Oral cephalexin is discontinued.

Six weeks later there is a significant reduction in the level of pruritus. The dog is mildly depressed and somnolent for 24 h after each treatment. There is early hair regrowth with follicular casts at the previously alopecic areas. Skin scrapes show low numbers of adult mites, both dead and alive. There are no immature stages or eggs. Treatment is changed to oral moxidectin, initially at 100 μg kg^{-1} day, increasing by 100 μg kg^{-1} day until a dose of 400 μg kg^{-1} day is reached.

Eight weeks later the dog is mildly pruritic, has good hair regrowth and no apparent skin lesions. Deep skin scrapes from the face and feet show no *Demodex*. Treatment is continued.

Six weeks later the dog is lesion free and non-pruritic. No mites are found on deep skin scrapes from the face, feet and lateral hind limbs. Medication is continued for 4 weeks then stopped.

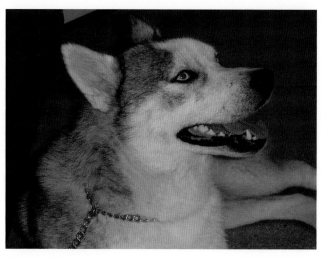

Figure 27.9 Shows the dog 5 months after initial presentation. There is complete resolution of the clinical signs. The dog has a bright (and less approachable!) demeanour.

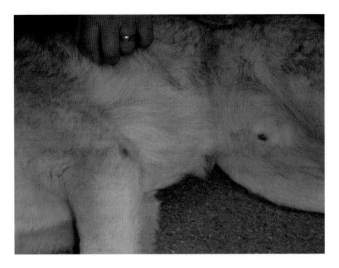

Figure 27.10 Shows the left lateral torso and groin. There is good new hair regrowth at the previously affected areas.

Prognosis

The prognosis is fair. The dog responds well to treatment, but there is a small risk of recurrent disease and the need for ongoing therapy.

Discussion

Demodex canis is a normal commensal of dogs that have had physical contact with their mother. Mites transfer from dam to pup in the first few days of life. Suggested factors predisposing to the overpopulation of *Demodex* mites include a genetic predisposition, poor nutrition, oestrus, endoparasites, stress and debilitating disease. This dog, at 1 year of age, had had three previous owners, a period in a rehoming kennels and was underweight at acquisition. The administration of glucocorticoids is also likely to have facilitated the disease.

Uncomplicated demodicosis is usually a non-pruritic condition. This dog had severe and sustained pruritus, probably due to the concurrent bacterial folliculitis.

Topical chlorhexidine was used initially to address the superficial bacterial pyoderma. Chlorhexidine is a good topical antibacterial choice. It has a residual action after rinsing, as it binds to the keratin of the skin surface. Benzoyl peroxide shampoo is also antimicrobial and has a good degreasing action. Used prior to amitraz treatment, benzoyl peroxide helps to increase exposure of the *Demodex* down the hair follicle to the amitraz applied on the skin surface.

Products licensed for the treatment of demodicosis in the United Kingdom are spot-on pipettes containing imidacloprid and moxidectin, or sarolaner, or amitraz solution diluted to a 0.05% concentration. This case was treated before the isoxazoline drug family became commercially available. An isoxazoline would now be an effective choice in such a case, due to the long duration of action and high efficacy in treating generalised demodicosis. Sarolaner is the only isoxazoline currently licensed in the UK for the treatment of demodicosis. An oral and systemic formulation of an isoxazoline is particularly useful when treating a plush-coated breed such as this Husky. Sarolaner can be used from 8 weeks of age and when the dog is over 1.3 kg in weight.

The imidacloprid and moxidectin spot-on was initially chosen because the dog had open wounds and there was a history of persistent diarrhoea concurrent with previous amitraz administration. The application of amitraz rinse to broken skin may have caused discomfort and unpredictable drug absorption. There are also practical difficulties when using topical wash treatments with plush-coated breeds. Diarrhoea is a recognised adverse reaction to amitraz along with vomiting, lethargy and depression of the central nervous system. Amitraz should not be used in pregnant or lactating bitches, diabetic animals or Chihuahuas.

There was only a modest reduction in mite numbers after six weekly applications of imidacloprid/moxidectin. The data sheet recommends a single dose every 4 weeks for 2–4 months in mild to moderate cases but states that, in severe cases, the product 'can be applied once a week and for a prolonged time'. A study compared the efficacy of an imidacloprid/moxidectin spot-on with an ivermectin positive control, in dogs with generalised demodicosis. The imidacloprid/moxidectin spot-on was given every 1, 2 or 4 weeks. The reduction in number of total live adult mites was 89, 64 and 45% in the groups with spot-on given every 1, 2 and 4 weeks, respectively. The group given ivermectin at 500 µg kg^{-1} by mouth once daily had a 98% reduction in the number of total live adult mites.

A good reduction in mite numbers was seen after 6 weeks of amitraz treatment. Diarrhoea was not seen during the second amitraz treatment, so the initial episode may have been unrelated to medication, especially as amitraz was originally used at half the current concentration for a suspected *Sarcoptes* infestation (0.025%). Depression and sleepiness were seen for 24 h after each amitraz rinse, probably due to alpha-2-adrenoreceptor agonist activity of the drug. Such adverse effects can be reversed by giving atipamezole or yohimbine. Injectable atipamezole can be given intramuscularly at the dose recommended for reversing medetomidine sedation. Dogs that show sedation after initial amitraz dips will not necessarily be sedated by the subsequent ones.

Oral milbemycin oxime is licensed, in combination with praziquantel, as an oral anthelmintic for dogs. It would have been the next choice under the prescribing cascade system for treatment of this case. However, the relatively high cost of daily treatment in this medium sized dog precluded its use. Oral moxidectin, another milbemycin of the macrocyclic lactone family, was introduced gradually while closely monitoring the dog. Ataxia, vomiting and lethargy have been reported as individual idiosyncratic and dose dependent adverse reactions to moxidectin.

Treatment was continued until two consecutive skin scrapes showed no *Demodex* mites. Therapy for generalised demodicosis is considered successful if there is no recurrence of clinical signs 1 year after stopping therapy. This dog has been in remission for several years.

Further reading

Ferrer, L., Ravera, I., and Silbermayr, K. (2014). Immunology and pathogenesis of canine demodicosis. *Veterinary Dermatology* 25: 427–435.

Fourie, J.J., Liebenberg, J.E., Horak, I.G. et al. (2015). Efficacy of orally administered fluralaner (Bravecto) or topically applied imidacloprid/moxidectin (Advocate) against generalised demodicosis in dogs. *Parasites and Vectors* 8: 187–193.

Greve, J.H. and Gaafer, S.M. (1966). Natural transmission of *Demodex canis* in dogs. *Journal of the American Veterinary Medical Association* 148: 1043–1045.

Mueller, R.S. (2011). Treatment of demodicosis in dogs: 2011 clinical practice. *Veterinary Dermatology* 23: 86–96.

Paterson, T.E., Halliwell, R.E., Fields, P.J. et al. (2009). Treatment of canine-generalized demodicosis: a blind, randomized clinical trial comparing the efficacy of Advocate* (Bayer Animal Health) with ivermectin. *Veterinary Dermatology* 20: 447–455.

Wagner, R. and Wendlberger, U. (2000). Field efficacy of moxidectin in dogs and rabbits naturally infested with *Sarcoptes* spp., *Demodex* spp. and *Psoroptes* spp. mites. *Veterinary Parasitology* 93: 149–158.

SECTION E

Ulceration

An *ulcer* occurs when a defined area of dermis is exposed and the overlying epidermis is absent. An ulcer is a deep lesion with exposed blood vessels, and has a tendency to bleed readily and to exude clear or haemorrhagic fluid. If the fluid is not licked or wiped away it will dry on the skin surface to form crust, which is found adjacent to or overlying the ulcer. Healing tends to result in scar formation because of the deficit in the dermis.

Ulcers form in a variety of ways, for example, following forceful skin trauma that breaches the resilience of the epidermis. This trauma can be self-inflicted and severe in response to focal irritation, such as with acral lick lesions in dogs or with allergic dermatitis in cats. Partial thickness skin trauma can also occur with road traffic accidents, caustic chemicals or thermal burns.

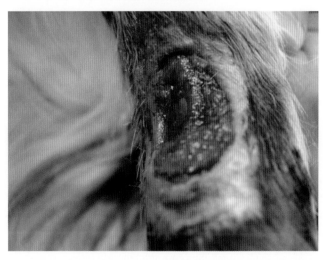

Figure E.1 Shows the flexor aspect of the left hock of a 3 year-old English Springer spaniel. There is an extensive deep ulcer filled with mature granulation tissue and surrounded by inflamed skin. The medial aspect of the ulcer has a deep section extending down to the exposed flexor tendon. This ulcer is self-inflicted and had progressed over a 10-month period despite symptomatic therapy. Radiographs showed degenerative joint disease restricted to this joint. The ulcer resolved with non-steroidal anti-inflammatories, appropriate exercise and wound care and environmental enrichment for the dog.

Ulceration can result from disruptions to the local blood supply of the skin. Vasculitis/vasculopathy usually affects a focal network of blood vessels and the skin normally supplied by those vessels can become devitalised and slough to leave an ulcer. The ulcers associated with larger vessel vasculitis are often circular and well defined and have a 'punched out' appearance.

The vesicles and bullae associated with certain immune-mediated diseases have their origins at the junction between the epidermis and the dermis. When a bullous lesion ruptures the epidermis is lifted away leaving an ulcer; for example, in bullous pemphigoid and epidermolysis bullosa.

Small Animal Dermatology: What's Your Diagnosis? First Edition. Jane Coatesworth.
© 2019 John Wiley & Sons, Inc. Published 2019 by John Wiley & Sons, Inc.

Focal inflammation of the skin can lead to ulceration. The inflammation is often organised in a nodular or diffuse pattern and made up of infiltrating neutrophils and macrophages. Inflammation can be triggered by infectious agents in the skin such as bacteria, fungi, *Leishmania* spp. and *Herpes* or pox virus. Ulceration is the second most common clinical skin sign of leishmaniosis, after exfoliative dermatitis and typically affects the pads and/or the ears. Alternatively, the inflammation that leads to ulceration may be a response to a spider or insect bite, or to a foreign body such as a grass seed. In calcinosis cutis, the body can mount an intense inflammatory response to calcium deposits in the skin, and attempts to extrude the calcium to the outside.

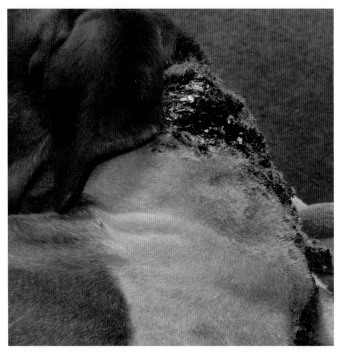

Figure E.2 Shows the dorsal neck of a 9 month-old Rhodesian Ridgeback. The dog is subdued and the neck area is painful, but the owners have not witnessed any rubbing or scratching of the area. There is an area of ulceration, approximately 12 cm in diameter, at the rostral end of the dorsal neck. The ulcerated area is wet with exudate and partially overlain with crust. A large dried crust is lifted away from the skin surface towards the caudal part of the dorsal neck. A broad band of erythema surrounds the crusted and ulcerated midline lesions. The dog was diagnosed with sterile immune-mediated meningitis and polyarthritis 2 months ago and given immunosuppressive doses of prednisolone. These calcinosis cutis lesions started 9 days ago and have progressed rapidly since.

Ulceration can occur in allergic skin disease, such as with an indolent ulcer on the lip of a cat. Ulcers may also be a sign of neoplasia, such as in squamous cell carcinoma.

Erosions are superficial lesions that only extend into the layers of the epidermis and do not breach the basement membrane. The epidermis does not contain blood vessels so erosions do not bleed. Erosions may have overlying crust from the dried content of a ruptured vesicle or pustule. Healing is by epithelial migration from the edges of the deficit and does not result in scar formation.

Erosions can have different underlying causes. The pustules of bacterial superficial pyoderma or pemphigus foliaceus form within the superficial layers of the epidermis. When the roof of a pustule ruptures a focal erosion remains. A focal area of epidermis can be abraded by mild to moderate self-excoriation such as in pyotraumatic dermatitis ('hot spot').

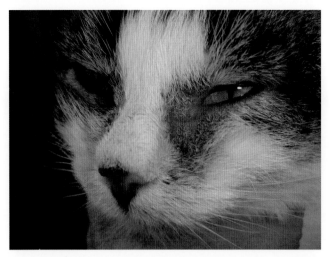

Figure E.3 Shows the face of a 3 year-old domestic shorthair cat. There is a small area of erosion at the medial canthus of the right eye, and a more extensive area adjacent to the left eye. The cat has atopic dermatitis, which is moderately well controlled with oral glucocorticoids. Cytology from the facial lesions shows a neutrophilic exudate with low numbers of extracellular cocci and high numbers of *Malassezia*.

Pseudomonas aeruginosa is an opportunistic pathogen of inflamed ears and skin, especially where the application of systemic or topical antimicrobials has already removed the resident microbial population. *Pseudomonas* spp. release a range of toxins and lytic enzymes that can damage the epidermis and cause erosive lesions.

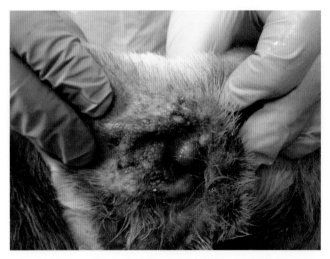

Figure E.4 Shows the right ear of a 9 year-old cross breed with untreated hypothyroidism. The dog has had recurrent episodes of staphylococcal otitis externa, has received multiple courses of antimicrobial ear drops and now has a multi-resistant *Pseudomonas aeruginosa* otitis externa. There is epithelial erosion of the length of the ear canal, including the external section visible here. The skin of the pinna and adjacent to the ear is thickened and hyperpigmented in keeping with the chronicity of the skin condition. The yellow/green purulent material coating the hairs around the ear is typical of *Pseudomonas*.

Strictly speaking, a sinus tract and a fistula are different things, even though the words are often used in a loose and interchangeable way. A *sinus tract* is blind ended and has one opening; for example, leading from deeply infected skin to the skin surface. In contrast, a *fistula* is a tract with two openings; for example, between an anal sac and the skin surface in a case of perianal furunculosis. Both sinus tracts and fistulae commonly open onto the skin surface in areas of ulceration. The presence of draining sinus tracts suggests that the deep layers of the skin are compromised; for example, in vasculitis, German Shepherd dog pyoderma and panniculitis.

History

A 13 year-old male, neutered English Springer spaniel presents with a 6-week history of discharging sinuses. Lesions were first noticed over the dorsal shoulders and at the left jugular region. The owner describes a large plum-sized lump appearing over the shoulders and rupturing the next day to produce a pale pink discharge. Multiple lumps of various sizes subsequently appeared over the trunk and rump, and rupture to produce variable amounts of discharge. The owner describes the dog as subdued and having a reduced appetite since the skin problem began. He is licking at the accessible discharging areas. He fell into a ditch containing a lot of brambles (*Rubus fruticosus*) 2 weeks before the first skin mass was noticed. The owner checked the dog for thorns at the time and he appeared unharmed other than a few superficial skin scratches. The dog has had more than 1 month of treatment with oral antibiotics with no improvement and has oral meloxicam long term for stiffness and suspected degenerative joint disease.

Questions

1. Describe the abnormalities and pertinent normal features in Figures 28.1–28.4.
2. What differential diagnoses should be considered for this presentation?
3. What tests could you perform to make the diagnosis?

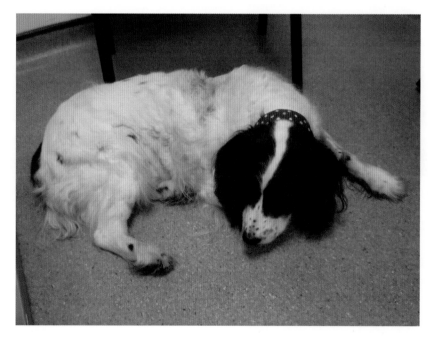

Figure 28.1

Small Animal Dermatology: What's Your Diagnosis? First Edition. Jane Coatesworth.
© 2019 John Wiley & Sons, Inc. Published 2019 by John Wiley & Sons, Inc.

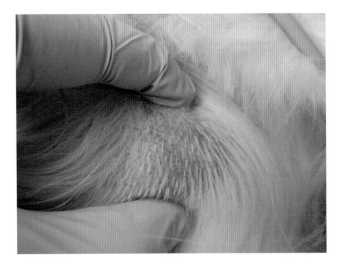

Figure 28.2

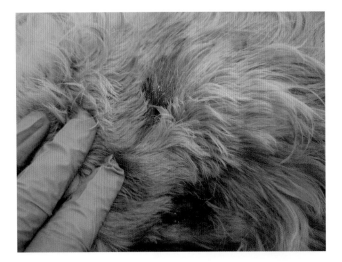

Figure 28.3

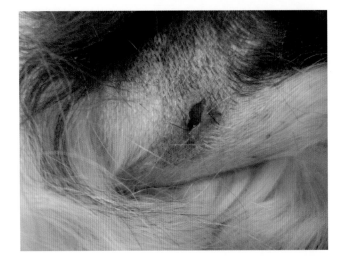

Figure 28.4

Answers

1. What the figures show

Figure 28.1 shows the dog during the initial consultation. He is subdued and lethargic, and spends the consultation lying on the floor. Some areas of hair coat have been clipped to remove dried exudate and matted hair, and to allow assessment of the skin lesions.

Figure 28.2 shows the right lateral thorax. There is a firm deep seated nodule, approximately 2.5 cm in diameter. The hair coat has been clipped to show the nodule and the mild erythema of the overlying skin. The dog shows signs of discomfort when the nodules are palpated.

Figure 28.3 shows two discharging sinuses over the dorsal shoulder region. The discharge has a clear to pink, glistening and slightly oily appearance. The surrounding hair coat is partially matted with crust. The sinuses are approximately 0.5 cm in diameter and the surrounding skin is swollen and erythematous.

Figure 28.4 shows the ventral abdomen. There is a well-demarcated deep ulcer with exudation. The surrounding hair coat has been clipped away. The ulcerated lesion measures 1.2 × 0.5 cm and is discharging a clear, slightly oily fluid. The skin adjacent to the ulcer is swollen and erythematous.

2. Differential diagnoses

Given the appearance of the skin lesions the following conditions should be considered:

- Sterile pyogranuloma/granuloma syndrome. This uncommon condition can present with nodules that ulcerate, but it does not form discharging sinuses and commonly involves the face.
- Neoplasia commonly forms masses deep in the skin. There may be ulceration to the skin surface if the centre of the mass is anoxic and becomes necrotic. This is more commonly seen in large tumours with an insufficient blood supply, and would be unusual in association with multiple small masses.
- Panniculitis can be sterile or have an infectious cause, and can be localised or multifocal. Localised panniculitis can usually be associated with foreign bodies, local trauma or injection site reactions. This case has multifocal lesions so infectious, systemic or immune mediated causes are more likely.

Sterile causes of panniculitis
Sterile nodular (immune mediated) panniculitis can present as a single nodule, or with multifocal lesions. The condition can be idiopathic, or associated with the following:

Injection site reactions.
Trauma.
Foreign body granulomas, perhaps around bramble thorns from the ditch
Secondary to pancreatic disease, for example to pancreatic neoplasia or pancreatitis. This rare form of panniculitis is mostly reported in Cocker Spaniels and has a distinctive histopathological appearance.

Infectious causes of panniculitis
Deep bacterial infections, including *Mycobacteria*, *Nocardia* and *Actinomyces*
Deep fungal infections
Protozoal infections (rare)

3. Appropriate diagnostic tests

Physical examination shows a subdued dog with an elevated rectal temperature of 40°C. The abdomen is tense on palpation and the dogs' stance is a little tucked. The owner feels he has lost weight, but no previous weight has been recorded for comparison.

Dermatological examination shows approximately 30 nodules and/or discharging sinuses distributed over the trunk, neck, rump, perineum and tail. No lesions are found on the head or the legs. The nodules, which are deep seated, measure 1–3 cm in diameter. A 1 cm wide × 6 cm long ulcer is located on the ventrolateral neck. This deep ulcer appears to have formed by a number of sinuses coalescing.

Cytology of some sinus discharge shows occasional red blood cells and no bacteria.

Haematology shows a leucocytosis 22.7×10^9 l^{-1} ($6–18 \times 10^9$ l^{-1}), mild neutrophilia 16.2×10^9 l^{-1} ($4–12 \times 10^9$ l^{-1}), lymphopenia 0.68×10^9 l^{-1} ($1–4.8 \times 10^9$ l^{-1}), monocytosis 2.95×10^9 l^{-1} ($0.1–1.8 \times 10^9$ l^{-1}) and eosinophilia 2.95×10^9 l^{-1} ($0.2–1.2 \times 10^9$ l^{-1}). The classic 'stress leukogram' of neutrophilia, lymphopenia and monocytosis is usually accompanied by an eosinopenia and is a response to exogenous or endogenous corticosteroids. The pattern here, including an eosinophilia, is more suggestive of chronic tissue damage and/or a purulent process, or the concurrent presence of parasites.

Serum biochemistry is unremarkable.

Skin biopsies are important to confirm the clinical suspicion of panniculitis and to look for potential underlying causes. Two small non-ulcerated nodules are excised intact for histopathology. It is important to go deep and to harvest the subcutis. Touch preparations are made onto clean glass slides for cytology from the deep margin of the fresh biopsy samples. These can be helpful in identifying bacteria or fungi. Both nodules are placed in formalin solution for histopathology. A third nodule is excised, the intact epidermis is cut away and the deep tissue is submitted for aerobic and anaerobic bacterial culture and sensitivity and fungal culture. Skin biopsy is recommended for a diagnosis of sterile nodular panniculitis (SNP), as the results of fine needle aspirates from nodules may be inconclusive or misleading.

There is no growth on aerobic or anaerobic bacterial or fungal culture and no micro-organisms are seen on cytology from the deep margin of the skin biopsies.

The histopathological appearance is similar for the two samples and shows a nodular pattern based in the subcutis and extending to the mid dermis. The nodules are composed of high numbers of macrophages and neutrophils and fewer lymphocytes. Special stains for fungi and bacteria, including acid fast bacteria, are negative and no foreign body material is seen.

Abdominal ultrasound shows a hypoechoic mass in the left mid abdomen. The mass measures 4.5×3.5 cm, has irregular margins and is surrounded by a marked focal mesenteric reaction. It is not possible to accurately define the origin of the mass. The mass could be arising from mesentery, large intestine, small intestine, metastasis or lymph node, but the location makes it unlikely to be from the pancreas. There are two well-defined nodules in the left liver lobes. They measure 5 and 7 mm in diameter and are hyperechoic in comparison to the surrounding parenchyma. These could represent nodular hyperplasia or neoplasia. There is a single, 5 mm diameter, hypoechoic nodule in the body of the spleen, which could be nodular hyperplasia, extramedullary haematopoiesis or neoplasia. The owner declined further investigation of the abdominal findings.

Thoracic radiographs show no obvious lung lesions. There is marked bridging ventral spondylosis of the thoracic and cranial lumbar vertebrae.

Diagnosis

Sterile nodular panniculitis. This case may be idiopathic, or may be associated with the abdominal changes that were seen on diagnostic imaging but that were not further characterised. Multifocal trauma, at the time of the fall into the ditch, is a possible underlying cause. Foreign body reactions to multiple penetrating bramble thorns was considered, but rejected as there is no evidence of plant material from the draining tracts or on histopathology.

Treatment

The oral meloxicam is stopped 2 days before starting treatment with prednisolone at 2 mg kg^{-1} given once daily with food. Vitamin E, 400 iu every 12 h, is given on an empty stomach. The skin is gently cleaned around the sinus tracts on a daily basis to reduce the likelihood of secondary bacterial infection and to maintain the dog's comfort.

Prognosis

The prognosis is difficult to quantify in this case as the nature and significance of the abdominal masses are unknown. The prognosis also depends on the response to treatment. If the dog has idiopathic SNP, unrelated to the abdominal findings, the prognosis is fair.

Further treatment and outcome

After 12 days of treatment the dog is much brighter, with more energy and improved exercise tolerance. No new nodules have appeared since starting the therapy. The numerous existing lesions are dry, with overlying crusts. The dose of prednisolone is reduced to 2 and $1 \, \text{mg kg}^{-1}$ on alternate mornings.

After a further 2 weeks of treatment the dog is bright and playful. There is moderate polyuria, polydipsia and polyphagia. There are multifocal circular plaques of granulation tissue at the site of the previous lesions. No new lesions have occurred. The prednisolone is reduced to $2 \, \text{mg kg}^{-1}$ every other day for 2 weeks, then $1 \, \text{mg kg}^{-1}$ every other day for 2 weeks, then $0.5 \, \text{mg kg}^{-1}$ every other day for 2 weeks and stopped. Oral ciclosporin is started at $5 \, \text{mg kg}^{-1}$ once daily. Ciclosporin is contraindicated in patients with a history of neoplasia, and the potential risks and benefits of this drug are discussed with the owner.

Seven weeks later all of the skin lesions have healed and no new lesions have occurred. There is a moderate amount of hair regrowth at the areas of clipped coat. The dog has had an occasional day when he is subdued and has a reduced appetite, but is otherwise bright and playful. There is no gastrointestinal upset with the ciclosporin.

Three months later the dog is acutely unable to stand on the hind limbs and is put to sleep.

Discussion

Panniculitis is an inflammation of the subcutis, the layer between the dermis and the muscular/fascial layers. The sub cutis is composed of variable amounts of subcutaneous fat, depending on the location and the condition score of the animal. It is usually the thickest layer of the skin. The subcutis also contains the panniculus muscle, blood vessels and connective tissue that gives structure to the lobules of fat.

Damaged fat cells release lipid, which is partially broken down to fatty acids. Both free lipids and fatty acids promote a significant inflammatory reaction and can lead to sterile granulomas. Idiopathic SNP is most commonly seen in Poodles and Dachshunds, but is a rare condition and the detailed patho-mechanism is not understood. There is no gender or age predisposition.

The largest lesion in this case, and the last to heal, was a $1 \times 6 \, \text{cm}$ deep slit-like lesion on the ventrolateral neck. The neck is a common lesion location, along with the abdomen and chest, although lesions can occur at any site. In common with other immune mediated conditions the lesions have a tendency to wax and wane. The onset of an active lesional phase can be accompanied by pyrexia and lethargy. In this case, the owner commented during treatment that the dog was more active and playful. This may be due to the lesions regressing, and/or to the wider analgesic and anti-inflammatory effects of glucocorticoids in this older dog.

Single or small numbers of nodules can be excised, but there is a risk of further nodules occurring. Topical dexamethasone ointment applied once daily to clipped skin, or intra-lesional dexamethasone, has been reported as an effective treatment option when only one or two nodules are present. However, most cases of SNP present with multiple nodules and need systemic treatment. This case went into complete remission with prednisolone and vitamin E, and was transitioned to ciclosporin to mitigate the adverse effects of the glucocorticoids. It is possible that either prednisolone or vitamin E may have been effective as sole treatments. Other treatment options include oral tetracycline/niacinamide, prednisolone/azathioprine or oral potassium iodide.

Further reading

Contreary, C.L., Outerbridge, C.A., Affolter, V.K. et al. (2015). Canine sterile nodular panniculitis: a retrospective study of 39 dogs. *Veterinary Dermatology* 26: 451–464.

Kim, H.J., Kang, M.H., Kim, J.H. et al. (2011). Sterile panniculitis in dogs: new diagnostic findings and alternative treatments. *Veterinary Dermatology* 22: 352–359.

O'Kell, A.L., Inteeworn, N., Diaz, S.F. et al. (2010). Canine sterile nodular panniculitis: a retrospective study of 14 cases. *Journal of Veterinary Internal Medicine* 24: 278–284.

History

A 2 year-old male neutered Japanese Akita is presented with a 3-month history of pedal discomfort. The owner initially reported a puncture wound on the haired skin of the left hind limb, proximal to the metatarsal pad and presumed to be caused by trauma. The dog licks at the affected area and is intermittently lame on the left hind limb. The dog was aggressive when the affected paw was handled, and was treated with systemic antibiotics and non-steroidal anti-inflammatory drugs. There was no improvement with the treatment and the persistent tract was explored, under general anaesthesia, with forceps and flushing. No foreign body was found. About 1 month after the first occurrence, a similar lesion appeared on the right hind limb. The dog was treated with prednisolone, at $1\,mg\,kg^{-1}$ once daily for 6 weeks. Both lesions resolved, along with the associated discomfort, but they recurred when the dose of prednisolone was tapered.

Questions

1. Describe the abnormalities and pertinent normal features in Figure 29.1.
2. What differential diagnoses should be considered for this presentation?
3. What tests could you perform to make the diagnosis?

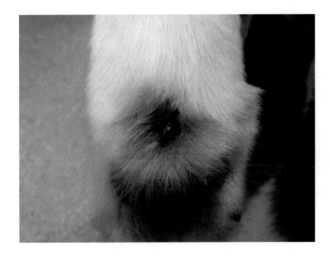

Figure 29.1

Answers

1. **What the figures show**

   Figure 29.1 shows the plantar aspect of the left hind limb. There is a well-defined sinus approximately 1 cm proximal to the metatarsal pad and in the midline. The sinus is 7 mm in diameter and discharging a small amount of clear fluid. The surrounding hair is matted with dried exudate and discoloured. A matching lesion (not shown) is present on the right hind foot.

Small Animal Dermatology: What's Your Diagnosis? First Edition. Jane Coatesworth.
© 2019 John Wiley & Sons, Inc. Published 2019 by John Wiley & Sons, Inc.

2. **Differential diagnoses**

   Given the appearance of the skin lesions the following conditions should be considered:

- Metatarsal fistulation.
- Discharging sinuses due to foreign bodies or infectious agents would be very unusual in such a bilaterally symmetrical pattern and would not be expected to resolve completely after treatment with corticosteroids.

3. **Appropriate diagnostic tests**

   Biopsy of the lesion classically shows marked inflammation of the subcutis and may involve the overlying deep dermis. The lesions are a focal sterile panniculitis and appear similar on histopathology to panniculitis caused by deeply penetrating foreign bodies or deep bacterial or fungal infections. The characteristic restricted location, the appearance and behaviour and no history of external trauma are important pieces of information for the histopathologist. Deep wedge biopsies, rather than punch biopsies, are good sampling techniques for suspected panniculitis as the deep skin and subcutis needs to be harvested. Wound healing in this mobile area can be more difficult when the lesions are very close to the pad. Biopsies were not performed in this case as the lesions were classical for the condition, the lesions had shown a typical response to treatment and there was no history of external trauma.

Diagnosis

Presumed metatarsal fistulation.

Treatment

Medical treatment options include systemic corticosteroids, ciclosporin or Vitamin E, and topical 0.1% tacrolimus. Vitamin E can be given either with or without corticosteroids. Surgical excision is usually followed by the formation of recurrent lesions within weeks of the surgery. Monitoring is also an option if the dog has no associated clinical signs, as spontaneous resolution without treatment has been reported.

   This dog showed a recurrence of clinical signs when the dose of prednisolone was tapered below 1 mg kg^{-1} day. A dose of 1 mg kg^{-1} day is likely to be associated with adverse effects in the medium to long term, so other options were considered preferable. Ciclosporin, at 5 mg kg^{-1} once daily, was dispensed for systemic therapy. The dog had intermittent soft motions while on ciclosporin. After 6 weeks of treatment the sinuses had completed healed. The dog paid no attention to the areas and allowed the owner to handle the feet.

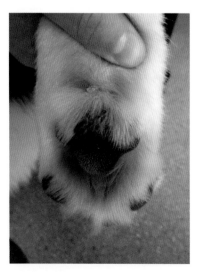

Figure 29.2 Shows the left hind limb after 6 weeks of ciclosporin treatment. There is a small circular crust overlying the skin. Removal of this crust shows that the sinus has completely healed. A thin cord of fibrous tissue is evident on palpation. The hair is returning to a more normal colour.

After 10 weeks of treatment, the frequency of ciclosporin was reduced to alternate day therapy and the owner was asked to apply topical tacrolimus once daily to the affected areas. Oral ciclosporin was stopped after 4 months and topical tacrolimus was continued on a twice-weekly basis. An owner should wear gloves when applying tacrolimus.

Prognosis

The prognosis is good, if ongoing treatment is well tolerated. The dog has had no recurrence after 1 year and tolerates the topical treatment well. The owner clips a small patch of hair away on a regular basis, with scissors, for ease of application of the cream.

Discussion

Metatarsal fistulation was first described in 1992, and was initially recognised in the German Shepherd dog. Despite the name of the condition, lesions can also be seen proximal to the carpal pads. This case shows the typical bilaterally symmetrical and midline location of the sinuses, but they may present with an asymmetric pattern and affect only one limb. The sinuses in this case are on the plantar metatarsal skin. A more common location would be on the haired skin immediately adjacent to the metatarsal pad. Sinus tracts can be single or multiple on any one leg.

German Shepherd dogs are the most commonly reported breed with this condition. Other reported affected breeds include the Weimaraner, Greyhound, Rottweiler and German Shepherd crossbreds. All of the reported cases are adult at the onset of clinical signs and are predominantly male.

Gastrointestinal signs are common in dogs receiving ciclosporin. Signs range from repeated vomiting and diarrhoea to mild inappetence and, as in this case, intermittent soft motions. One analysis of over 600 atopic dogs treated with ciclosporin showed that 25% developed vomiting and 18% developed soft stools or diarrhoea. These signs were mostly mild and transient and only a small percentage of dogs needed to stop the treatment. Maximal drug absorption is achieved by giving the drug on an empty stomach, however, gastrointestinal signs may be reduced by giving ciclosporin with food and the degree of bioavailability is only slightly reduced. Giving ciclosporin as a pre-measured frozen dose can also reduce the frequency of vomiting.

Metatarsal fistulation can go into remission with topical 0.1% tacrolimus alone. Topical treatment is not a suitable initial choice for this dog as he is aggressive, and presumably painful, when the hind paws have active lesions and are handled. Once the lesions have resolved with systemic treatment, the dog tolerates topical maintenance therapy with tacrolimus.

The lesions seen here are, strictly speaking, sinuses rather than fistulae but the term metatarsal fistulation has become an accepted title for this condition. The aetiology of the condition is not understood.

Further reading

Oliveira, A.M., Obwolo, M.J., van den Broek, A.H.M., and Thoday, K.L. (2007). Focal metatarsal sinus tracts in a Weimaraner successfully managed with ciclosporin. *Journal of Small Animal Practice* 48: 161–164.

Paterson, S. (1995). Sterile idiopathic pedal panniculitis in the German shepherd dog – clinical presentation and response to treatment of four cases. *Journal of Small Animal Practice* 36: 498–501.

Scholz, F., Muse, R., and Burrows, A.K. (2015). Focal metatarsal fistulae affecting a greyhound dog successfully treated with topical 0.1% tacrolimus ointment. *Veterinary Dermatology* 26: 488–490.

Steffan, J., Favrot, C., and Mueller, R. (2006). A systematic review and meta-analysis of the efficacy and safety of cyclosporin for the treatment of atopic dermatitis in dogs. *Veterinary Dermatology* 17: 3–16.

History

A 5 year-old male neutered German Shepherd dog presents with a 2-month history of straining and discomfort when passing faeces. The degree of discomfort has progressed over the past 2 weeks and there is now severe pain associated with defaecation. The dog shows signs of distress, physical tension and loud vocalisation around each episode of defaecation. Faeces are being passed 4–5 times each day. The faeces vary in consistency from liquid diarrhoea to soft formed motions. They have a yellow to brown colour and intermittently have additional fresh blood and/or mucous. The dog is unwilling to adopt a sitting posture and will either stand or lie down. The tail is held clamped down over the perineum. There are frequent and prolonged episodes of licking at the perineal area, including during the consultation. The dog is lethargic, has a variable appetite and has lost around 4 kg of bodyweight. The owners have noticed a novel and unpleasant odour over the past few weeks and feel that this is associated with one of the dogs. The other dog in the household is well and shows no clinical signs. There have been recent episodes of aggression between the two dogs while they are usually friendly and mutually tolerant. Both dogs are fed a commercial complete chicken-based dry food.

Questions
1. Describe the abnormalities and pertinent normal features in Figures 30.1 and 30.2.
2. What differential diagnoses should be considered for this presentation?
3. What tests could you perform to make the diagnosis?

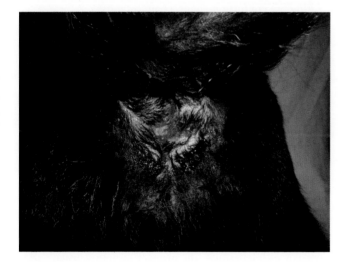

Figure 30.1

Small Animal Dermatology: What's Your Diagnosis? First Edition. Jane Coatesworth.
© 2019 John Wiley & Sons, Inc. Published 2019 by John Wiley & Sons, Inc.

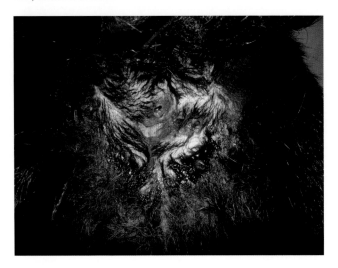

Figure 30.2

Answers

1. What the figures show

Figure 30.1 shows the perianal area with the tail elevated. The overlying matted hair coat has been partially clipped away to show the skin. There is a thick dark brown gelatinous discharge covering the clipped skin and matting the adjacent hair coat of the perineum and ventral tail. Note the low angle of tail elevation as, even with the dog sedated, lifting the tail further elicits a pain response.

Figure 30.2 shows a closer view of the perianal area with the tail elevated. The skin is wet and the area is malodorous. There is a thin trail of yellowish liquid faeces just below the anus. There are three large ulcerated areas, one above the anus and two to the right of the anus. The one above the anus has a small slit-like ulcer to the right. Each ulcer is surrounded by a ring of grey and devitalised skin that will subsequently slough to leave a large confluent area of ulceration.

2. Differential diagnoses

Given the appearance of the skin lesions the following conditions should be considered:

- Perianal furunculosis. The clinical signs, and the breed, are typical for this condition.
- Anal sac abscessation and subsequent rupture. The presence of an abscess can be painful, especially just prior to and at the time of rupture. Abscessation can be associated with focal licking and regional discomfort, however, the associated pain is usually diminished once the abscess drains and the pressure is relieved.
- Concurrent inflammatory bowel disease (IBD) with either of the mentioned conditions.
- Dogs with anal sac adenocarcinoma can present with tenesmus. The primary tumour is usually unilateral and rounded, and occurs at over 10 years of age. There may be asymmetrical swelling in the perianal area, but not ulceration. Hypercalcaemia is a paraneoplastic syndrome seen in 25–50% of dogs with anal sac adenocarcinoma. Lethargy, depression and poor appetite can be seen with hypercalcaemia, but polyuria and polydipsia will commonly accompany these signs.

3. Appropriate diagnostic tests

General *physical examination* shows a restless, anxious and underweight dog (30 kg). The perianal region is examined under sedation as the dog is very painful in this area. The dense hair coat is clipped away from the perianal area and from the proximo-ventral tail. The hair overlying the perineum is wet and matted with a malodorous tenacious dark brown discharge.

Palpation of the perianal region shows diffuse inflammation of the right upper quadrant. The three sinus tracts can be probed to a depth of 0.5–1.3 cm. The tracts are blind ended and do not have connection to the rectum or the anal sacs.

Palpation of the anal sacs per rectum shows that both sacs have a smooth rounded and distinct outline. The sacs are moderately full and the contents, which have a normal appearance, can be expressed with gentle pressure. The contents discharge onto the skin surface through their ducts that are close to, but separate from, the ulcerated areas. Palpation of the empty anal sacs reveals a normal flat and flaccid area with no nodules or thickening suggestive of neoplasia.

Diagnosis

Perianal furunculosis. The diagnosis is based on the compatible history and clinical signs, and the typical breed. The anal sacs are normal in this case. There is possible concurrent IBD.

Treatment

A low residue novel protein diet is recommended to reduce the frequency of defaecation and to support any concurrent IBD. The dog is fed a commercial hydrolysed dry diet. The diet is approximately 90% digestible and contains soy, which is a novel protein source for this dog. Normally, a 2-week food trial is recommended to investigate the possibility of a concurrent food-responsive IBD. However, this dog is in significant discomfort so immunomodulatory treatment is started straight away. Such treatment is likely to have a positive effect on both IBD and perianal furunculosis.

Oral ciclosporin is given at 5 mg kg^{-1} once daily. The dog vomits repeatedly within 20 min of the medication being given, this is repeated on several occasions. The measured aliquot of liquid ciclosporin is frozen in an ice cube tray before administration and there is no further vomiting.

Oral prednisolone, at 1 mg kg^{-1} once daily with food, is given for the first week of treatment to give some symptomatic relief in this very uncomfortable dog.

After the first week of treatment the dog is more relaxed and comfortable, and the owner is able to clean the perianal area daily with a hypochlorous acid solution. The cleaning is facilitated by keeping the hair coat cut short around the anus and the ventral tail.

Prognosis

The prognosis is fair. The dog has made a good initial response to treatment, but relapses can occur. A good long-term outcome is dependent on a continued response to treatment, the maintenance of an appropriate dose of drug therapy, limited adverse effects to therapy and limited progression of inter-current disease such as IBD.

Further treatment and outcome

After 1 month of treatment, the lesions have healed and the dog is comfortable and relaxed.

Attempts to reduce the dose of ciclosporin below 2.5 mg kg^{-1} once daily result in recurrence of early lesions and associated licking of the perineum. Intermittent scavenging of meat protein appears to trigger diarrhoea and flatulence. The dog is maintained on ciclosporin and a hydrolysed soy diet for 3 years, he is comfortable and has a stable bodyweight.

Discussion

Perianal furunculosis is very largely a disease of the German Shepherd dog and occurs in adult dogs of any age. Despite a strong breed predilection, the genetic basis for the disease has not been fully elucidated. This may be because both genetic and environmental factors are at play in the development of the condition.

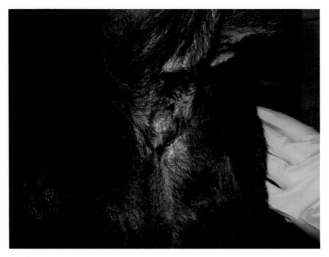

Figure 30.3 Shows the perianal area after 1 month of treatment. The dog is not sedated and is much more comfortable and relaxed with the tail held elevated to examine the area. There is hair regrowth at the previously clipped areas. The skin has healed in the areas that were ulcerated. There is a thin layer of liquid yellowish faeces covering the perianal skin.

The pathogenesis of perianal furunculosis is not completely understood, but it is considered to be an immune mediated disease. German Shepherd dogs appear to have deficiencies in some of the immune defence mechanisms that are normally active at the skin and mucosal surfaces. These include impaired mucosal barrier function and impaired immunological tolerance to normal bacteria and/or food allergens in the gut. Immune surveillance, with appropriate recognition and processing of 'self and other', is very important at the outer boundaries of the body including the gut, skin and nasal passages. Diseases such as IBD, idiopathic deep pyoderma, aspergillosis and perianal furunculosis may result from inadequate innate immunity at the mucosal or skin surfaces. The German Shepherd dog is over-represented in all of these diseases.

This case shows many of the typical features of perianal furunculosis. There is a chronic and progressive disease course, the dog strains to defaecate, has pain on defaecation and has blood in the stools. There is also anorexia, weight loss and a depressed demeanour. The lesions extend approximately 120° around the anus, but some cases can completely surround the anal ring.

The anal sacs have a variable degree of involvement in perianal furunculosis. They may be normal and unaffected, may be inflamed, have fistulae extending from the sac to the rectum or extending from the sac to the perianal skin. Careful palpation of the sacs and probing of the open tracts can help to understand the extent and distribution of the disease.

Oral ciclosporin is considered to be the primary treatment option for perianal furunculosis. The generally good clinical response to this T lymphocyte modulating drug gives support to the theory of an immune mediated pathogenesis for the disease. Ciclosporin is not licensed for the treatment of perianal furunculosis and needs informed owner consent. Prior to the availability of ciclosporin, cases were treated with immunosuppressive doses of prednisolone, either alone or with the addition of azathioprine, and overall response rates were less favourable. Prednisolone $\pm$ azathioprine is a useful treatment option if treatment with ciclosporin is unsuitable or ineffective. Short-term prednisolone can give rapid symptomatic relief, as in this case, during the first week or two of ciclosporin treatment.

This case responds to the relatively low ciclosporin dose of 5 mg kg^{-1} once daily. The extent and severity of the lesions and the degree of discomfort typically improve in the first few weeks of treatment. If there is an inadequate response after 8 weeks of treatment the dose can be increased to 7.5 mg kg^{-1} once daily or 5 mg kg^{-1} twice daily. High doses of ciclosporin are costly for a large breed like a German Shepherd dog. Ciclosporin can be given concurrently with ketoconazole to make treatment more affordable, but care needs to be taken to avoid ketoconazole toxicity. Ketoconazole is a triazole antifungal drug that inhibits cytochrome P450 enzyme activity. Ciclosporin is largely metabolised by this enzyme system in the liver, so the addition of ketoconazole potentiates the available dose of ciclosporin. Various dose combinations are described including 2.5 mg kg^{-1} of ciclosporin and ketoconazole once daily, 5 mg kg^{-1} of ciclosporin and ketoconazole once daily, and 1 mg kg^{-1} of ciclosporin with 10 mg kg^{-1} ketoconazole once daily.

Tacrolimus is another calcineurin inhibitor and has a similar mode of action to ciclosporin. Cases can be transitioned onto topical tacrolimus cream as a maintenance therapy. The 0.1% cream is applied intermittently to the perianal skin at the lowest frequency that prevents the recurrence of lesions. People can experience a burning or tingling sensation at the site of tacrolimus application and the same effect may occur in a proportion of dogs.

Surgical intervention can be helpful after medical therapy for the removal of persistent sinus tracts and/or involved anal sacs. Surgery can be followed by anal stenosis or the recurrence of the lesions. Faecal incontinence can occur if there is surgical damage to the nerves of the anal sphincter or the sphincter itself. Flatulence may result from a reduction in anal sphincter tone. The perianal area has a good blood supply for wound healing, but persistent contamination of the region by faecal material increases the risk of wound breakdown after surgery.

Further reading

Doust, R., Griffiths, L.G., and Sullivan, M. (2003). Evaluation of once daily treatment with cyclosporine for anal furunculosis in dogs. *Veterinary Record* 152: 225–229.

Hardie, R.J., Gregory, S.P., Tomlin, J. et al. (2005). Cyclosporine treatment of anal furunculosis in 26 dogs. *Journal of Small Animal Practice* 46: 3–9.

Jamieson, P.M., Simpson, J.W., Kirbyand, B.M., and Else, R.W. (2002). Association between anal furunculosis and colitis in the dog: preliminary observations. *Journal of Small Animal Practice* 43: 109–114.

History

A 3 year-old female neutered Border Collie presents with a history of skin ulceration in both axillae. The lesions first appeared 10 months ago and have waxed and waned in severity since that time. During the past month, similar ulcerated lesions have occurred in the groin. The regular application of topical fusidic acid/dexamethasone gel brings improvement, but not resolution and the condition quickly relapses on stopping therapy. The dog licks persistently at the lesions and sometimes wears an Elizabethan collar to prevent licking. Despite the lesions being present in frictional areas the dog is very active and keen to exercise.

Questions

1. Describe the abnormalities and pertinent normal features in Figures 31.1–31.3.
2. What differential diagnoses should be considered for this presentation?
3. What tests could you perform to make the diagnosis?

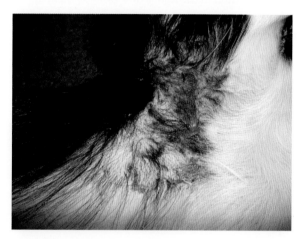

Figure 31.1

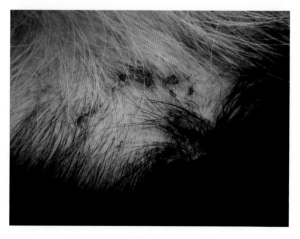

Figure 31.2

Small Animal Dermatology: What's Your Diagnosis? First Edition. Jane Coatesworth.
© 2019 John Wiley & Sons, Inc. Published 2019 by John Wiley & Sons, Inc.

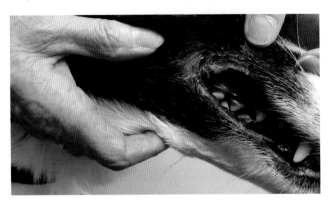

Figure 31.3

Answers

1. What the figures show

Figure 31.1 shows well demarcated areas of active ulceration in the right axilla. Both pigmented and non-pigmented skin is affected. There is a copious amount of exudate from the lesions. Some of the exudate has dried to form a crust, which is matted into the hair coat both overlying and adjacent to the ulcers. The left axilla is similarly affected.

Figure 31.2 shows a cluster of ulcers in the left groin. The ulcers at the top of the photograph form an undulating line, typical of the disease. These lesions are healing. They have a rim of erythema and swelling associated with inflammation, and are contracting in size as they heal. The ulcers are smaller in size than the axillary lesions and have less associated exudation and crust. Both images were taken on the same day and show different stages of ulceration in the different locations.

Figure 31.3 shows the right side of the mouth. There is focal ulceration of the caudal half of the upper lip margin and around the commissure of the lips. The left side of the mouth is similarly affected.

2. Differential diagnoses

Given the appearance of the skin lesions the following conditions should be considered:

- Vesicular cutaneous lupus erythematosus (VCLE)
- Erythema multiforme
- Lupus-like drug eruption.

3. Appropriate diagnostic tests

Physical examination is unremarkable.

Dermatological examination shows ulcerated lesions in the axillae, groin and at the lip margins, with a bilaterally symmetrical distribution. The ulceration in the axillae is active, exudative and associated with overlying and adjacent crust. The lesions in the groin are healing.

Skin biopsies. Given the possibility of a lupus type condition there is a risk of tissue shearing at the interface between the dermis and the epidermis. Delicate tissue handling and a biopsy technique that avoids twisting the tissue are helpful to produce optimal samples. Elliptical biopsies were taken with a scalpel blade, rather than punch biopsies taken using a circular biopsy punch. The inclusion of very early erythematous lesions and the erythematous margins of early ulcerated lesions improves the likelihood of seeing active primary pathology and of making a definitive diagnosis.

The histopathology shows multifocal ulceration with proliferation of fibrovascular granulation tissue in the ulcerated defects and numerous neutrophils at the ulcerated surface mixed with necrotic tissue. There is moderate to prominent vacuolation and apoptosis of the basal keratinocytes. An inflammatory infiltrate, rich in lymphocytes and plasma cells, significantly obscures the interface between the epidermis and the dermis. This histological pattern supports the clinical suspicion of VCLE.

Diagnosis

Vesicular cutaneous lupus erythematosus (VCLE).

Treatment

Avoid unnecessary exposure to ultraviolet light. The owner does not exercise the dog in the middle of the day during the summer months. The dog wears a sun suit, during the summer months, when participating in outdoor agility competitions. The material of the suit blocks ultraviolet light. The cut is modified to avoid any pressure on the axillae and groin, and to allow maximum ventilation for this highly active dog.

Immunomodulation. The dog is given a combination of oral niacinamide (500 mg every 8 h), oxytetracycline (500 mg every 8 h) and essential fatty acid supplementation. The matted hair is gently clipped away from the affected skin and many of the crusts come away with the hair coat. Tacrolimus is applied in a thin layer to the affected skin once daily with a gloved finger, reducing to alternate day application after 4 weeks.

After 8 weeks of treatment the areas of ulceration in the axillae and lip margins have largely healed. A few 2 mm diameter new crusted lesions, with underlying ulceration, are noted in the groin. Oral prednisolone is added at 0.5 mg kg^{-1} every other morning with food. The dog is bright and well, has much reduced licking of the affected skin and has resumed agility training. Topical tacrolimus is reduced to twice-weekly application.

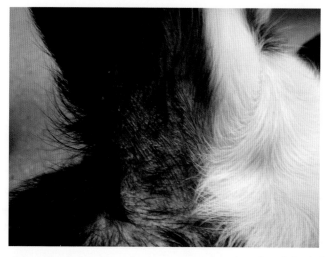

Figure 31.4 Shows the right axilla after 8 weeks of treatment. The ulcers have largely healed. There is a vertical line of adherent crust overlying the site of the formerly most ulcerated area. The exposed skin of the medial antebrachium is thin, wrinkled and inelastic, probably associated with the previous repeated application of topical dexamethasone.

After a further 10 weeks of treatment all of the ulceration has resolved and there have been no new lesions for the past 5 weeks. The owner has discontinued topical therapy. There are multifocal circular or oval alopecic and hyperpigmented areas in the axillae and groin at the sites of previous ulceration.

After a further three months of treatment the dog is doing well and oxytetracycline is discontinued.

The owner applies topical tacrolimus for a few days at the earliest sign of new lesions occurring and the lesions do not progress. Oral prednisolone is reduced to 0.3 mg kg^{-1} every other day.

Prognosis

Good, if the lesions respond well to treatment and the treatment is well tolerated by the dog.

Final outcome

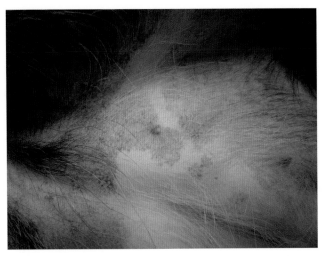

Figure 31.5 Shows the skin of the groin after 2 years of treatment. There are subtle changes in pigmentation at the previously affected sites, but otherwise the skin is robust and free of lesions.

This dog has been monitored for 4 years since diagnosis and is receiving niacinamide, essential fatty acid supplementation, low dose alternate day prednisolone and occasional topical tacrolimus. The observant and motivated owner checks the dog regularly and sees a new lesion starting in the axillae or groin on an occasional basis. Physical examination shows an occasional small hyperpigmented macule in these areas.

Discussion

This condition was initially described as an ulcerative dermatosis affecting the Rough Collie and the Shetland Sheepdog. More recently it has been recognised in the Border Collie and in crosses featuring one of the three affected breeds. Adult dogs can become affected at any age, with the disease often starting during the months with maximum levels of ultraviolet light. Cases in the Border Collie may have a less severe phenotype and respond well to lower levels of medication.

VCLE is part of the cutaneous lupus erythematosus family of diseases. These diseases have characteristic histopathological findings of a lymphocyte-rich interface dermatitis, apoptosis and vacuolation of the basal keratinocytes and inflammation of the epidermis and superficial dermis. In VCLE the dying basal keratinocytes form a cleft between the epidermis and the dermis, resulting in a vesicle. The vesicles rapidly rupture to leave areas of ulceration.

This case shows a typical distribution of ulceration at the axillae, groin and lip margins. The ventral abdomen, medial thighs, oral cavity, anus, vulva, periocular skin and concave surfaces of the pinnae can also be affected. The lesions take the form of single or co-joined rings and undulating lines, and may merge to form extensive areas of ulceration. Secondary bacterial infections may complicate the disease and require the gentle application of topical anti-microbial treatment, with or without systemic antibiotics.

Topical tacrolimus is licensed for the treatment of moderate to severe atopic dermatitis in people, and is unlicensed in the dog. It is available at concentrations of 0.03–0.1%. Tacrolimus, like ciclosporin, is in the calcineurin inhibitor drug family. It works as a potent inhibitor of T cells, a helpful mode of action for this lymphocyte mediated disease. Approximately 50% of people report some skin sensation, such as tingling, warmth or burning, after the topical application of tacrolimus. The skin irritation is usually of mild to moderate severity and tends to resolve within 1 week of starting treatment. Owners need to monitor their dog for signs of possible discomfort after the treatment is applied.

This dog was successfully treated with a combination of oxytetracycline, niacinamide and topical tacrolimus. Oxytetracycline, including the alternatives tetracycline or doxycycline, along with niacinamide have a range of immunomodulatory and anti-inflammatory actions. The dose of tetracycline/niacinamide was originally described as 250 mg of each drug, given every 8 h, for dogs under 10 kg, and 500 mg of each drug every 8 h for dogs over 10 kg. Adverse effects to the drug combination are uncommon, but some dogs have lethargy, vomiting, diarrhoea and/or inappetence. Giving the drugs with food or stopping only the niacinamide may resolve the adverse effects. The tetracycline antibiotics are readily bound by cations and their absorption will be much reduced if they are given with rich sources of iron, magnesium, aluminium, zinc or calcium, including dairy products and some antacids. Other reported treatment options for VCLE include systemic ciclosporin, and immunosuppressive doses of prednisolone or methylprednisolone, either alone or in combination with azathioprine.

Further reading

Banovic, F., Robson, D., Linek, M., and Olivry, T. (2017). Therapeutic effectiveness of calcineurin inhibitors in canine VCLE. *Veterinary Dermatology* 28: 493–498.

Font, A., Bardagi, M., Mascort, J., and Fondevila, D. (2006). Treatment with oral ciclosporin A of a case of VCLE in a rough collie. *Veterinary Dermatology* 17: 440–442.

Gibson, I. and Barnes, J. (2011). VCLE in a Border Collie in New Zealand. *New Zealand Veterinary Journal* 59: 153.

Jackson, H.A. and Olivry, T. (2001). Ulcerative dermatosis of the Shetland sheepdog and rough collie may represent a novel vesicular variant of CLE. *Veterinary Dermatology* 12: 19–27.

Lehner, G.M. and Linek, M. (2013). A case of VCLE in a Border Collie successfully treated with topical tacrolimus and nicotinamide-tetracycline. *Veterinary Dermatology* 24: 639.

White, S.D., Rosychuk, R.A., Reinke, S.I., and Paradis, M. (1992). Use of tetracycline and niacinamide for treatment of autoimmune skin disease in 31 dogs. *Journal of the American Veterinary Medical Association* 200: 1497–1500.

History

An adult entire male Staffordshire Bull Terrier cross, of unknown age, is picked up a few days earlier wandering the city streets as a stray. The dog has no collar or microchip and the rehoming charity is unable to find an owner, or anyone who recognises the dog. During the few days at the rehoming centre the dog is subdued, has a normal appetite and thirst, and appears to be healthy other than having skin lesions. The dog is not showing any pruritic behaviour.

Questions

1. Describe the abnormalities and pertinent normal features in Figures 32.1–32.3.
2. What differential diagnoses should be considered for this presentation?
3. What tests could you perform to make the diagnosis?

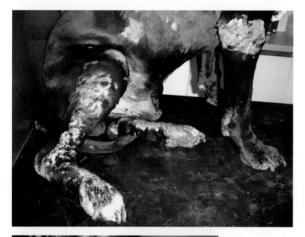

Figure 32.1

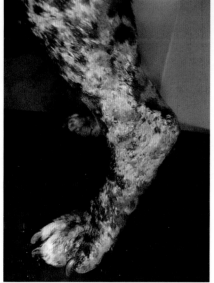

Figure 32.2

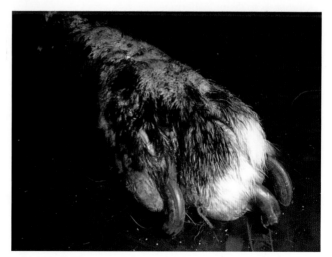

Figure 32.3

Small Animal Dermatology: What's Your Diagnosis? First Edition. Jane Coatesworth.
© 2019 John Wiley & Sons, Inc. Published 2019 by John Wiley & Sons, Inc.

Answers

1. What the figures show

Figure 32.1 shows the lower right side of the body. There are large patches of alopecia and erythema on the lateral elbow, lateral body wall, caudal to the right carpus and on both hind limbs from the stifle down. Small areas of hair loss are seen on the tail. The remaining hair coat has a normal glossy appearance.

Figure 32.2 shows the lateral aspect of the lower left hind limb and some of the right hind paw. There is extensive alopecia and marked erythema. The affected skin is thickened with an uneven surface contour. There are multifocal sinus tracts draining haemorrhagic fluid onto the skin surface. Some discrete deep skin nodules are palpable proximally, but more distally there is a confluent thickened plaque over the lateral hock.

Figure 32.3 shows more detail of the swollen right hind paw. There is tight apposition between the swollen digits and serosanguinous fluid oozes from the skin when the dog moves. The nails are long, typical of a dog with chronic pododermatitis.

2. Differential diagnoses

Given the appearance of the skin lesions the following conditions should be considered:

- Deep bacterial pyoderma
- Deep fungal infection
- Neutrophilic folliculitis and furunculosis (Sweet's syndrome)
- Eosinophilic folliculitis and furunculosis (Well's syndrome)

Underlying causes of deep bacterial pyoderma:
Demodicosis
Endocrinopathies, such as hypothyroidism or hyperadrenocorticism. The age of this dog is unknown but it is likely to be middle-aged or older.
Chronic treatment with immunosuppressive drugs. This dog has an unknown history, so the possibility of previous treatment should be considered.
Chronic allergic skin disease. The skin barrier function in this type of disease is compromised by self-trauma and/or by innate structural defects. Compromise of the barrier function predisposes to secondary bacterial infection, initially in the form of surface or superficial bacterial pyoderma that can progress to deep pyoderma.
Less common bacterial types, for example *Nocardia*, *Actinomyces* and *Mycobacteria*.

3. Appropriate diagnostic tests

General physical examination is unremarkable other than marked enlargement of the prescapular and popliteal lymph nodes. The dog appears to be subdued and fearful, but there is no known range of normal behaviour to compare this with.

Dermatological examination shows extensive skin lesions on all four limbs and fewer changes on the lateral body wall and tail. The head, upper trunk and ventral abdomen have no skin lesions.

Cytology. An impression smear is obtained by cleaning the skin over a sinus tract and then squeezing the skin to express fluid from the deeper tissue. An alternative sampling method is to take a fine needle aspirate from an intact skin nodule. The smear is dried, stained and examined under the microscope. There are numerous neutrophils and macrophages. The absence of visible bacteria in the sample does not exclude a diagnosis of deep pyoderma.

Hair plucks and deep skin scrapes do not demonstrate any *Demodex* mites.

Haematology and serum biochemistry are unremarkable. Alterations in these values may suggest an inter-current disease either related or unrelated to the skin signs, or an adverse effect of previous medication.

Skin biopsy for bacterial culture and sensitivity. The aim of skin biopsy for tissue culture is to isolate the micro-organisms from the deep tissue, without contamination from the inevitable surface population.

The hair is clipped away and the skin surface prepared as for sterile surgery. The surface of the skin needs to be dry before the biopsy is taken, to prevent antiseptic fluid from running down to the deeper tissues. The tissue culture returned a heavy growth of *Escherichia coli*, sensitive to a restricted number of antibiotics, including fluoroquinolones.

Skin biopsy for histopathology. Skin biopsies for histopathology benefit from minimal clipping and no scrubbing. This allows the surface skin layers, and any adherent material, to remain intact and to be available for the pathologist to examine. Full thickness biopsies are taken from nodular and inflamed areas, but avoiding sinus tracts and areas of ulceration, and using an 8 mm biopsy punch.

The histopathology shows a nodular and pyogranulomatous pattern. There are dense accumulations of neutrophils, with fewer macrophages and multinucleated giant cells, some of which have small fragments of keratin at the centre. Many of the hair follicles are partially or completely effaced by inflammatory cells.

No bacteria or fungal elements are identified on special stains.

Diagnosis

Bacterial deep pyoderma, with an unknown history and unknown underlying cause.

Treatment

Oral marbofloxacin is given once daily at $2\,mg\,kg^{-1}$ and the dog is bathed twice each week in a chlorhexidine-based shampoo. The dog is brighter and more active after 4 weeks of treatment and the skin is less swollen and erythematous.

Further diagnostic tests

A *blood sample* is taken for total T4 and TSH assay. The T4 result is in the low normal range and the TSH assay is normal, ruling out hypothyroidism.

A free catch *urine sample* has a urine cortisol: creatinine ratio in the normal range, ruling out a diagnosis of hyperadrenocorticism.

Both of these tests are intentionally delayed until the dog is clinically well and the skin infection is improving, as both tests can give false positive results when there is active inter-current disease.

Prognosis

The prognosis is fair as the deep bacterial pyoderma responds well to treatment, but the history and underlying cause is unknown and the condition may recur.

Discussion

Bacteria are less commonly seen on cytology from deep pyoderma lesions, in contrast to the common appearance of bacteria in samples from surface and superficial pyoderma. The ulcerated and crusted skin surface associated with deep pyoderma is a supportive environment for bacterial overgrowth, hence the value of surface cleaning before sampling or aspirating a sample from an intact nodule with a fine needle. Bacterial overgrowth usually presents with high numbers of extracellular bacteria on cytology, while bacterial pyoderma has intracytoplasmic bacteria inside neutrophils and/or macrophages.

Bacterial culture and sensitivity is recommended in all cases of deep bacterial pyoderma. While superficial pyoderma is commonly associated with *Staphylococcus pseudintermedius*, the bacterial species predominating in deep pyoderma is less predictable. Deep pyoderma often involves Gram negative rod-shaped bacteria, such as *Proteus*, *E. coli* and *Pseudomonas aeruginosa*, which have an inherently unpredictable sensitivity to antibiotics. Antibiotics to treat deep pyoderma are often given for months rather than weeks so for reasons of antibiotic stewardship, potential adverse reactions and cost it is important to select the appropriate antibiotic in the first instance.

Deep pyoderma occurs when infection is established in the dermis and/or the subcutis. This can occur locally when there is penetration of bacteria into the dermis following skin trauma, for example on a penetrating foreign body, during a road traffic accident or in a fight. Focal areas of deep pyoderma are also seen following the trauma of repeated pressure at elbow callouses, along the dorsum after inappropriate grooming techniques and after repeated self-trauma in acral lick granulomas. Deep pyoderma occurs following the rupture of hair follicles and the release of hair shaft fragments, skin cells and bacteria into the dermis. The contents of the hair follicle, which have previously been 'outside' of the body, are recognised as foreign bodies in the dermis and subcutis. The immune system mounts an inflammatory response and leads to the clinical signs of pain, swelling, erythema and heat. Other signs can include haemorrhagic bullae, draining sinus tracts, ulceration and dried crust. Pruritus is rarely a clinical feature of deep pyoderma. Chronic lesions may scar to leave firm, fibrosed and alopecic areas of skin.

A specific form of immune mediated deep pyoderma is seen in German Shepherd dogs and their crosses. Lesions tend to occur on the groin, trunk and lateral thighs. The affected skin forms a mosaic of hyperpigmented and ulcerated areas, with overlying crust and variable draining sinuses.

Further reading

Beco, L., Guaguère, E., Lorente Méndez, C. et al. (2013). Suggested guidelines for using systemic antimicrobials in bacterial skin infections: part 2 – antimicrobial choice, treatment regimes and compliance. *Veterinary Record* 172: 156–160.

History

A 5 year-old female entire Saint Bernard is presented with profuse bleeding from the nose. Bright red blood is spurting rhythmically from the centre of the nose, the owner is intermittently attempting to apply pressure but the dog resists this. A less severe episode of bleeding occurred 5 days ago and the dog was anaesthetised to investigate the affected area. The bleeding appeared to be coming from the nasal philtrum. A 2 mm punch biopsy was taken from this area. The biopsy site bled profusely, before a double layer closure and prolonged digital pressure arrested the bleeding. The owner reports that an ulcer on the nasal philtrum was first noticed 7 months earlier and has gradually enlarged. The dog does not show any signs of pruritus or pain associated with the lesion. The owner has applied a variety of emollient and occlusive topical products with no apparent effect, other than the dog wiping them away. The dog is otherwise well and has no apparent bleeding elsewhere on the body. There is no history of trauma and the dog had not received any drugs for 10 months before the nasal lesion was first noticed.

Questions

1. Describe the abnormalities and pertinent normal features in Figure 33.1.
2. What differential diagnoses should be considered for this presentation?
3. What tests could you perform to make the diagnosis?

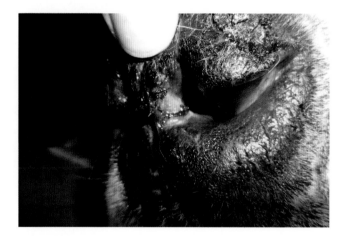

Figure 33.1

Answers

1. **What the figures show**

Figure 33.1 shows the nasal planum from the left. The philtrum is stretched dorsally by digital pressure to show the extent of the ulceration. The biopsy sites are sutured with two metric PDS. There is a single area of well-defined linear ulceration spanning the width of the nasal planum. The lesion is orientated at 90° to the nasal philtrum and is symmetrically distributed. The ulcer is relatively narrow at the base compared to the wide superficial opening, giving a V-shaped profile when seen from the side. The dorsal half of the nasal planum is hyperkeratotic.

Small Animal Dermatology: What's Your Diagnosis? First Edition. Jane Coatesworth.
© 2019 John Wiley & Sons, Inc. Published 2019 by John Wiley & Sons, Inc.

2. Differential diagnoses

Given the appearance of the skin lesions the following conditions should be considered:

- Arteritis of the nasal philtrum.
- A bleeding disorder. These can be primary, involving the blood vessel walls, platelets or platelet function or secondary involving problems with coagulation factors.
- Trauma to the nasal philtrum resulting in tissue loss and subsequent haemorrhage. The steady progression of the lesion over time and the absence of a history of trauma makes this less likely.
- Squamous cell carcinoma (an ulcerative form). The dog was initially referred to the oncology department for this possibility.
- Leishmaniosis.

3. Appropriate diagnostic tests

Haematology. The dog had an episode of bleeding 5 days ago and has a current arterial bleed.

There is a low haemoglobin $10\,g\,dl^{-1}$ (12–$18\,g\,dl^{-1}$), low red blood cell count $4.2 \times 10^{12}\,l^{-1}$ (5.5–$8.5 \times 10^{12}\,l^{-1}$) and low haematocrit $0.297\,l/l$ (0.37–$0.55\,l/l$). The elevated absolute reticulocyte count of $236.3 \times 10^9\,l^{-1}$ indicates a regenerative red blood cell response (regenerative when $>60 \times 10^9\,l^{-1}$). The blood smear shows slight polychromasia and an occasional nucleated red blood cell consistent with the release of immature red blood cells from the bone marrow.

Clotting profile. The prothrombin time (PT), activated partial thromboplastin time (APTT) and thrombin clot time (TCT) are all within normal limits.

Histopathology from the original 2 mm punch biopsy shows inflammation with neutrophils and lymphocytes, and no evidence of neoplasia. Further deep biopsies from the affected area show proliferation and thickening of arterial walls, and associated arterial stenosis in the deep dermis.

Diagnosis

Arteritis of the nasal philtrum.

Treatment

The dog is given oral oxytetracycline 500 mg every 8 h, niacinamide 500 mg every 8 hours, and hydrocortisone aceponate spray applied once daily using a soft swab.

After 4 weeks of treatment there has been no further bleeding. There is healthy granulation tissue at the base of the ulcer. Oxytetracycline and niacinamide are continued, and the frequency of topical hydrocortisone aceponate is reduced to twice weekly.

Three months later there has been no further bleeding and the dog has no apparent nasal discomfort. The deficit in the nasal philtrum is still present, but a rim of new epithelial cells is progressing from the ventral margin. The dog is lost to follow up after this.

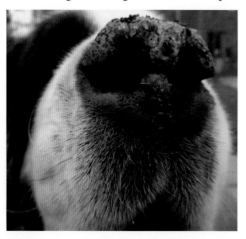

Figure 33.2 Shows the nasal planum after three months of treatment, on the same day as Figure 33.3. The base of the ulcer has a bed of granulation tissue, which has thickened to reduce the depth of the lesion.

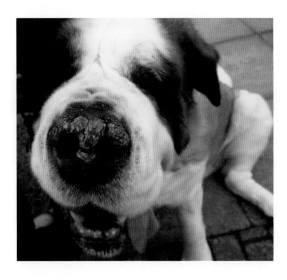

Figure 33.3 Shows the nasal planum after 3 months of treatment. There is a pale pink rim of new epithelial cells visible at the ventral border of the affected area.

Prognosis

The prognosis is good, if the medication is tolerated by the dog.

Discussion

This condition is visually distinctive and highly localised. It was first described in the literature in 2002 by Torres et al., affecting one Giant Schnauzer and three Saint Bernard dogs, a further affected Saint Bernard is described in the addendum. Since then, cases have been described in a Bassett Hound, a further Saint Bernard and a Newfoundland, and reported in a Labrador Retriever, further Saint Bernard dogs and a crossbreed dog. The onset of clinical signs is between 3 and 6 years of age. The frequent association with the Saint Bernard suggests a genetic component to the disease in this breed.

The proposed pathogenesis of this condition is a primary inflammation of the large vessels (arteries and arterioles) supplying the nasal philtrum. The walls of the vessels become thicker and restrict or occlude blood flow through the vessel lumen. The tissues of the central philtrum which are usually nourished by these blood vessels become hypoxic and die, leaving a large focal ulcer. The particular and diagnostic change seen in histopathology from skin biopsies is inflammation of the arteries of the deep dermis and of the arterioles immediately below the ulcer.

Medical treatment options described in the literature include oral prednisolone (1.1 mg kg^{-1} day) as monotherapy, in combination with topical gentamicin/betamethasone valerate, or in combination with systemic tetracycline/niacinamide and fish oil. Topical fluocinolone in dimethyl sulfoxide (DMSO) every 12 h has also been used as monotherapy. The clinical signs tend to relapse if medication is discontinued, but respond again to renewed treatment. This dog responded to a combination of oral niacinamide/oxytetracycline and topical hydrocortisone aceponate. The aim of long term medical treatment is to give the lowest dose of medication that prevents the recurrence of haemorrhage from the nasal philtrum.

A surgical treatment option is described in two dogs. The affected tissue of the nasal philtrum is resected and the arteries supplying the area are ligated before closing the deficit. One dog had no recurrence of clinical signs after 34 months of follow up. The second dog had recurrence of mild clinical signs after 4 years, and was controlled with topical 0.1% tacrolimus.

Further reading

Gross, T.L., Ihrke, P.J., Walder, E.J., and Affolter, V.K. (eds.) (2005). Proliferative arteritis of the nasal philtrum. In: *Skin Diseases of the Dog and Cat*, 2e, 255–256. Oxford, UK: Blackwell Science.

Pratschke, K.M. and Hill, P.B. (2009). Dermal arteritis of the nasal philtrum: surgery as an alternative to medical therapy in two dogs. *Journal of Small Animal Practice* 50: 99–103.

Torres, S., Brien, T.O., and Scott, D.W. (2002). Dermal arteritis of the nasal philtrum in a Giant Schnauzer and three Saint Bernard dogs. *Veterinary Dermatology* 13: 275–281.

History

A 10 month-old female entire Labrador Retriever presents with a history of sudden onset facial swelling. The swelling was first noticed at the left eyelid and the left side of the muzzle. The lesions progressed rapidly in extent and severity over the past 4 days. During this time the dog received antibiotics, opioid analgesia, anti-histamines and intravenous fluids. Discharging lesions developed over the muzzle and a swab was taken from the discharge for bacterial culture and sensitivity. The dog was vaccinated as a puppy, and given anthelmintics and flea control at the same time. The owner has two other dogs, neither of which are affected. The dog is subdued, but eating and drinking a normal amount.

Questions

1. Describe the abnormalities and pertinent normal features in Figures 34.1–34.4.
2. What differential diagnoses should be considered for this presentation?
3. What tests could you perform to make the diagnosis?

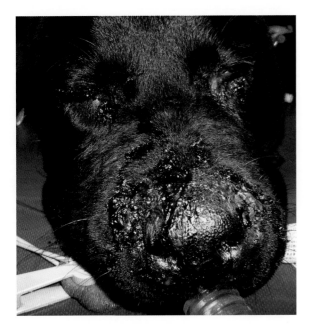

Figure 34.1

Small Animal Dermatology: What's Your Diagnosis? First Edition. Jane Coatesworth.
© 2019 John Wiley & Sons, Inc. Published 2019 by John Wiley & Sons, Inc.

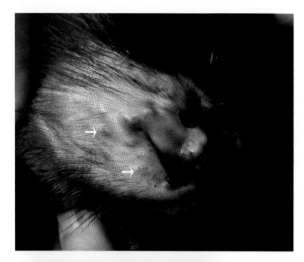

Figure 34.2

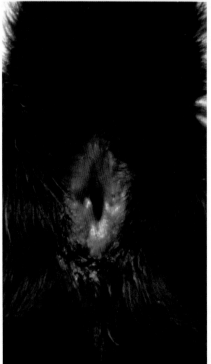

Figure 34.3

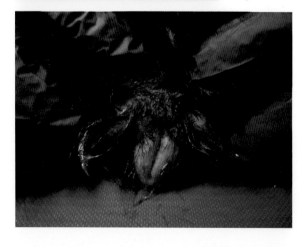

Figure 34.4

Answers

1. What the figures show

Figure 34.1 shows the dog's face, while under general anaesthesia. There is significant swelling of the muzzle and around the eyes. Both eyes have a yellow mucopurulent discharge, most apparent at the medial canthus of the left eye. There is multifocal skin ulceration around the eyes, along the bridge of the nose and at the rostral muzzle. There are multiple erythematous papules. Multiple sinus tracts are discharging a haemopurulent fluid, which has partially dried in some areas to form dark coloured crust.

Figure 34.2 shows the concave aspect of the right pinna. There are approximately a dozen firm nodules, each measuring 2–5 mm in diameter, in the sparsely haired area. The skin is intact over most of the nodules. The two nodules indicated by the white arrows have soft fluctuant points and thin overlying skin. The nodule at the bottom right has been recently abraded and has some fresh haemorrhage at the apex.

Figure 34.3 shows the anal area. There is erythema and diffuse swelling of the anal ring. There are also multifocal nodules around the anus, of between 3 and 5 mm in diameter.

Figure 34.4 shows the vulva. There is significant swelling and erythema of the vulval lips and the adjacent tissue of the vulval fold. The vulva is held everted from the vulval fold for the photograph. There is a copious amount of yellow purulent material coating the skin and hair.

2. Differential diagnoses

Given the appearance of the skin lesions the following conditions should be considered:

- Juvenile cellulitis
- Generalised demodicosis with secondary bacterial pyoderma
- Adverse drug reaction (the last known medication was an anthelmintic given 6 months ago)

3. Appropriate diagnostic tests

Physical examination shows a friendly and responsive, but depressed, dog. The oral mucous membranes are slightly reddened and swollen with a normal capillary refill time. The mandibular, prescapular and popliteal lymph nodes are all firm and markedly enlarged on palpation. The rectal temperature is mildly elevated (39.4°C). There is marked bilateral conjunctival hyperaemia. In addition to the skin changes shown in the figures, all of the nail beds are swollen and erythematous.

Cytology. Hair plucks from the rostral muzzle and periocular area show no *Demodex* mites.

An impression smear of the haemopurulent discharge from the rostral muzzle shows high numbers of non-degenerative neutrophils and no micro-organisms.

Skin biopsies. Full thickness skin biopsies are taken with a 6 mm biopsy punch from the dorsal and rostral muzzle, and dorsal to the vulva. Tissue is taken for histopathology using clean technique, and for deep tissue culture using sterile technique. Histopathology shows severe multifocal pyogranulomatous dermatitis and panniculitis, consistent with juvenile cellulitis. Special stains do not reveal any evidence of infectious agents. Bacterial culture of the deep biopsy tissue returns no aerobic or anaerobic bacterial growth. The bacterial culture results from the initial swab of facial discharge also return no bacterial growth.

Diagnosis

Juvenile cellulitis (also known as puppy pyoderma, puppy strangles, and juvenile sterile granulomatous dermatitis and lymphadenitis).

Treatment

Treatment is started with oral prednisolone, at 2 mg kg^{-1}, given in the morning with food.

After 48 hours the dog is brighter in demeanour and the skin lesions show no further progression.

After 2 weeks of treatment the dog is bright and alert. She tires quickly at exercise, has a slightly increased appetite and thirst and is urinating more frequently. All of these changes can be ascribed to her glucocorticoid medication. There is an area of thick crust on the dorsorostral muzzle. Gentle pressure over the crust produces a bead of pus from the proximal edge. An impression smear of this purulent material shows high numbers of neutrophils with intracytoplasmic cocci, consistent with a bacterial infection. The perianal and vulval areas show mild crusting and some alopecia. There is mild erythema and a small amount of crust on the periocular skin. The conjunctivae now have a normal appearance. The peripheral lymph nodes are slightly enlarged on palpation. The dog is eating well, but has lost 0.2 kg of bodyweight. The prednisolone is reduced to 1.75 mg kg^{-1} or 0.75 mg kg^{-1}, given once daily on alternate mornings for 10 days, and then further reduced to 1.75 mg kg^{-1} every other morning for 10 days. Oral potentiated amoxicillin is given, at 12.5 mg kg^{-1} every 12 hours, for a 3-week course.

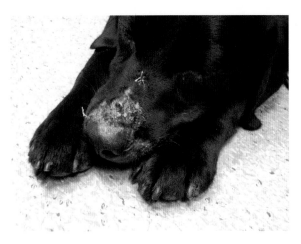

Figure 34.5 Shows the dog's face after 4 weeks of treatment. There is mild swelling and erythema of the rostral muzzle and periocular skin. A clearly demarcated area of alopecia is present around the nasal planum, with a large adherent crust to the left of the dorsal midline. Skin sutures, which are about to be removed, mark the healed skin biopsy sites.

After 5 weeks of treatment the swelling and erythema has largely resolved. The skin is dry and there are numerous crusts at the previously affected areas. A number of crusts have been shed and the underlying skin is dry. There is a small amount of crust on the dorsorostral aspect of the muzzle, but this is thin and starting to detach. The peripheral lymph nodes feel normal on palpation. The dog has lost a further 0.3 kg of bodyweight. The dose of prednisolone is reduced to 1.5 mg kg^{-1}, given every other morning with food for 2 weeks and then further reduced to 0.75 mg kg^{-1} every other morning for 2 weeks.

After 9 weeks of treatment the dog has a more normal appetite and thirst, and is urinating less frequently. She is brighter and able to maintain longer spells of exercise with a stable bodyweight. There is well demarcated multifocal alopecia on the concave aspects of the pinnae, dorsal to the vulva and surrounding the nasal planum. The dose of prednisolone is reduced to 0.5 mg kg^{-1} every other day for 2 weeks and then stopped.

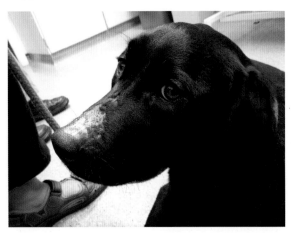

Figure 34.6 Shows the dog's face after 9 weeks of treatment. There is a large patch of well demarcated alopecia on the dorso-rostral muzzle and small patches of alopecia around the eyelid margins.

One month after stopping prednisolone the owner reports that the dog is bright and active, has gained a further 0.5 kg of bodyweight and has good exercise tolerance.

Prognosis

The prognosis is good, as the dog responds well to treatment and recurrence is unlikely.

Discussion

Juvenile cellulitis usually occurs in young dogs between 3 weeks and 4 months of age. This case was unusual in the later age of onset of 10 months, although there are a few published case reports of affected adult dogs. A wide range of breeds can be affected, but Golden Retrievers and Dachshunds are thought to be predisposed. A number of puppies in the same litter can be affected.

Swelling of the eyelids and lips, with enlargement of the submandibular lymph nodes, are the earliest and most common clinical signs. Affected lymph nodes may rupture and drain, hence the name 'puppy strangles'. (The equine disease 'strangles' can show rupture and drainage of the submandibular lymph nodes, but is a primary bacterial disease.) There is variable involvement of the pinnae, vulva, prepuce and anus. The involvement of the nailbeds was unusual in this case.

The pathogenesis of the disease is poorly understood. Bacterial involvement is secondary, making 'puppy pyoderma' a misnomer. The prompt and complete response to immunosuppressive doses of corticosteroids suggests an immune mediated mechanism. Although immunosuppression raises concerns in this young population of affected dogs, it is important to act decisively once the diagnosis is confirmed. Inadequate or delayed treatment can cause prolonged distress for the patient and lead to significant long-term scarring.

Further reading

Neuber, A.E., Broek, A.H.M., Brownstein, D. et al. (2004). Dermatitis and lymphadenitis resembling juvenile cellulitis in a four year old dog. *Journal of Small Animal Practice* 45: 254–258.

White, S.D., Rosychuk, R.A., Stewart, L.J. et al. (1989). Juvenile cellulitis in dogs: 15 cases (1979–1988). *Journal of the American Veterinary Medical Association* 195: 1609–1611.

Diagnosis by Case

Section A. **Alopecia**

Case 1. Hyperoestrogenism, associated with a retained testicle that has undergone neoplastic transformation

Case 2. Hypothyroidism with a secondary bacterial superficial pyoderma

Case 3. Flea bite hypersensitivity

Case 4. Sarcoptic mange

Case 5. Feline paraneoplastic alopecia

Case 6. Colour dilution alopecia

Case 7. Dermatophytosis

Case 8. Canine flank alopecia, iatrogenic hyperadrenocorticism and generalised demodicosis

Section B. **Pigmentation**

Case 9. Discoid lupus erythematosus

Case 10. Adult onset generalised demodicosis, with *Malassezia* dermatitis and bilateral *Malassezia* otitis

Case 11. Vitiligo

Case 12. Canine atopic dermatitis, with secondary bacterial superficial pyoderma, bacterial overgrowth and intertrigo.

Case 13. Uveodermatologic syndrome

Case 14. Epitheliotropic lymphoma

Section C. **Pruritus**

Case 15. Atopic-like dermatitis, with bacterial overgrowth and *Malassezia* overgrowth

Case 16. Sarcoptic mange

Case 17. Atopic dermatitis

Case 18. Eosinophilic folliculitis and furunculosis

Case 19. Pyotraumatic dermatitis

Case 20. Atopic-like dermatitis, with secondary superficial bacterial pyoderma and bilateral *Malassezia* otitis externa

Section D. **Pustules, crust and scale**

Case 21. Pemphigus foliaceus

Case 22. Sebaceous adenitis

Case 23. Cheyletiellosis

Case 24. Hepatocutaneous syndrome

Case 25. Dermatophytosis

Case 26. Pemphigus foliaceus

Case 27. Juvenile-onset generalised demodicosis with secondary bacterial folliculitis

Section E. **Ulceration**

Recommended Reading

Muller and Kirk's Small Animal Dermatology. Edited by Miller, Griffin and Campbell, and published by Elsevier. This book is considered by most to be the standard comprehensive textbook. The latest edition is the seventh, published in 2013. A weighty tome packed with useful information, arranged by the cause of the disease and well indexed to make the material readily accessible. The book has a North-American perspective.

Skin Diseases of the Dog and Cat: Clinical and Histopathologic Diagnosis. By Gross, Ihrke, Walder and Affolter, published by Blackwell Science in 2005. This excellent and unique book explains the clinical presentation and the histopathology of each condition. It gives clinicians a more thorough understanding of each disease process by relating the macroscopic to the microscopic. The book does not contain information on treatment.

Canine and Feline Skin Cytology by Francesco Albanese, published in 2016 by Springer International Publishing. This book contains lots of good quality photographs of inflammatory and neoplastic cytology, along with clear and helpful text. It is a useful text to keep close to the microscope.

Small Animal Dermatology: What's Your Diagnosis? First Edition. Jane Coatesworth.
© 2019 John Wiley & Sons, Inc. Published 2019 by John Wiley & Sons, Inc.

Index

Small Animal Dermatology: What's Your Diagnosis? First Edition. Jane Coatesworth.
© 2019 John Wiley & Sons, Inc. Published 2019 by John Wiley & Sons, Inc.